STRESSED IN

THE TRUTH ABOUT STRESS AND HOW TO RELEASE YOUR PERSONAL BARRIERS TO WELLNESS

Dr. Robert C. Bornstein

New Perspective Publishing
Malibu, California

STRESSED IN

New Perspective Publishing
All rights reserved.
Copyright © 2009 by Robert C. Bornstein

ISBN 978-0-9841-6950-4

No part of this book may be reproduced or transmitted in any form or by any means, electronic or mechanical, including photocopying, recording, or by any information storage and retrieval system, without permission in writing from the author. For information contact the author at www.stressedin.com.

Printed in the United States of America

This book is dedicated to everyone
who can acknowledge the truth
that we are all intricately connected,
and who have the courage
to live their life
with a resolute commitment
to beautify this connection.

CONTENTS

Chapter One	WELCOME TO YOUR NEIGHBORHOOD	1
Chapter Two	VISITORS WITH ATTITUDE	11
Chapter Three	THE SILENCE OF THE WAVES	25
Chapter Four	THE SLEEPERS MUST AWAKEN	45
Chapter Five	WAVES OF HUMANITY	49
Chapter Six	IT'S GETTING ON YOUR NERVES	91
Chapter Seven	GOOD VIBRATIONS	109
Chapter Eight	SPIRITUAL INFLUENCES	115
Chapter Nine	RELEASING STRINGS	123
Chapter Ten	THE VIBRATION OF DESIRE	129
Chapter Eleven	BUILDING A SOLID FOUNDATION	137
Chapter Twelve	THE BLOOD/BRAIN BARRIER TO WORLD HEALING	153
Chapter Thirteen	MY DOCTOR SAID	167
Chapter Fourteen	WE ARE ALL MENTORS AND STUDENTS	181
Chapter Fifteen	WELCOME HOME	185
Acknowledgments		187
About the Author		189

CHAPTER ONE

WELCOME TO YOUR NEIGHBORHOOD

You are about to embark on a unique journey. As you read and absorb the text, you will acquire keys that will enable you to approach your highest and best potential. You will learn the truth about stress and how stress energy is impacting your body health. You will discover that you have much more control over your health and well-being than you may have been led to believe. You may learn more about yourself and everyone in your life than you have ever known.

We are being swept into the twenty-first century on an exponentially expanding web of technology, including the World Wide Web. Unfortunately, many have decided to "live" there. Since you live within the fabric of a universe, and not on a web, it is vitally important that you acquire a clear understanding of how to navigate within the natural fabric and learn to wean yourself from the insidious stress-producing factors that invade your body space every second of every day. With this new foundation of knowledge, your ability to connect the dots for the highest benefit to you and to others will be greatly enhanced.

Stress manifests within to create a situation where your body is not at ease. The book will provide a blueprint that will enable you to identify, manage, and release the influences of stress energy. This in turn will unlock barriers to wellness. You will also learn how to optimally engage all of the natural healing energies and influences that are so vital to your well-being. You have the ability to tap into your body's highest potential. Somewhere along the way you may have forgotten how to use the keys.

It's time to refresh your memory…

We have arrived at an historically unprecedented crossroads where there is a true urgency for all of us to expand our knowledge of the energetic forces and influences that interact with our bodies. As you travel through the text, you will gain a clear understanding of the factors that have brought us to what can only be described as a tipping point. We have distanced ourselves so far from the rhythms of nature that we risk becoming critically "stressed-in." Does this sound unpleasant? It is. If you are one of the hundreds of millions of people around the world who can never seem to achieve a true state of ease, you can attest to the truth of this. To remedy this situation, we must accelerate the movement along our personal learning curves and help others to do the same. The good news is that your body is often much closer to returning to its natural state than you may have been led to believe.

Some of you say that you "feel fine" and believe that you are presently at your highest plateau of wellness. When your journey through the text is complete, you may see that this is just not the case, and you will understand that there are higher levels of wellness beyond your current framework of knowledge. Thus, for all of you, even those who have not manifested obvious symptoms, the knowledge presented is likely to be the most complete set of preventive care keys you have ever had within your grasp.

LET'S BEGIN!

*Societal influences have taught us to believe that
"What you see is what you stress."*

In other words, we have been led to believe that every challenging situation that occurs in a relationship, workplace, or other area of our life is to blame for our ills. Thus, we have become used to saying, "I'm stressed out." This is totally inaccurate. A more accurate term is "stressed-in." I will use this term throughout the text. Let's just say that from this moment on, if you choose to cling to the thought that life's challenges are the cause of stress, you are setting yourself up for much hardship.

Since few have ever been properly educated about the true nature of stress, isn't it ironic that the statements, "You need to get rid of your stress" or "You need to take care of your stress," are usually among the top ten list of words of advice given to us by concerned family, friends, and practitioners of the healing arts. How can you be expected to "get rid of" or "take care of" something when you don't know what it is in the first place? So, let's get right to the truth of the matter.

Stress occurs when:

Energy-in-motion disrupts the natural harmony of your body
at a quantum level,
forcing your body to expend energy and resources
to repair and recalibrate this imbalance.

When this continues on a chronic basis,
it results in persistent disharmony and energetic imbalance
within your body,
leading to a state where
your body is not at ease.

When your body is not at ease, every one of your cells becomes vulnerable to a state of inflammation, dysfunction, degeneration, or even transformation. Thus, the importance of acquiring a full set of keys to unlock any ongoing barriers to wellness.

Energy-in-motion comes in an ocean of "flavors." There are naturally good and restorative varieties, and then there are disruptive and hindering varieties. We are immersed in this sea and saturated by it. Realizing your highest potential depends on understanding the full spectrum of energy-in-motion and how it relates to your health. You will learn that **there is no neutral energy in your life.** There are obvious, and not so obvious, natural energies and influences that are omnipresent, purposeful and vital to your body health as long as you acquire knowledge of how to engage them properly; and then there are unnatural energetic influences that always stress you in. I am sure that you will not be too surprised when you learn that specific emotional energy-in-motion from your own mind is the most disruptive to your body, followed closely by the toxic by-products of shortsighted industrial and technological attempts to improve our lives.

A unique, but very common manifestation of stress also occurs when the body experiences a "disconnect" from loving influences. The understanding of what constitutes a true loving influence and how a "disconnect" usually occurs, will make all the difference in the world to your health and well-being.

As you travel through and absorb the text, you will also see that there is no "game of chance" when it comes to your body health or your life ongoing. You have much more control over the quality and longevity of your life than you may have been led to believe. Hence, **there is no luck.** Luck lies in the realm of randomness, chance, and false assumptions. On the other hand, good energetic influences always allow you to be at your best, which gives you access to the most favorable outcomes! In fact, it is more thoughtful if you substitute the phrase "good energy" whenever you think of saying, "good luck."

Having an intimate understanding of your body's building blocks will provide the knowledge that will motivate you to show the highest respect for your body and the bodies of others. Thus, let's begin with the building blocks of what you are made of…your neighborhood within…as I will refer to your body. As you will soon see, if you visualize and refer to your body as your neighborhood, you will be more likely to give it the respect it deserves by keeping it as peaceful and pristine as possible. I guarantee that your body will love you for it!

Your Neighborhood 101

Don't panic. Although your neighborhood does have a quantum flavor, this is not a physics course. You will be given the facts you need to understand the true nature of your body, and, I promise, you will only have to know one short equation. In fact, let's begin with that equation.

You should all be familiar with Einstein's: $E = mc^2$

> E is **energy**
>
> m is the **mass** of something. Since we are talking about your body, let's call **m** the "matter," or "stuff," that your body is composed of.
>
> c^2 is **a very large number** that is constant. (For those who like more detail, it's the natural velocity of light energy squared – approximately 300,000,000 meters per second squared!)

Thus, energy = the stuff, or matter, you are made of, multiplied by a huge number, and, as you will soon learn, everything you do, say, or think does matter! In essence, then, you are energy… and a lot of it.

In fact, you have more energetic potential than you could possibly imagine – a virtual ocean of energy units called joules (pronounced like jewels). You can realize this potential only if you choose to apply the knowledge that you are about to acquire.

The stuff you are made of

If you could break down your entire body into the smallest of building blocks, you would discover that you are made of quarks and electrons. Yes, even your DNA is made of these tiny particles. It may not sound glamorous, but that's the way it is. To be more specific, the quarks make up the centers (or nuclei) of all of your atoms, and the electrons race around the quarks. What is really interesting is that if we could take all of the individual quarks and electrons in your body and total up their individual masses, we would measure just a very small percentage of your expected number of pounds!

Where is all of the other mass? For the answer we have to look at your quirky quarks. It just so happens that they never like to be alone, so they prefer to hang out in threes. (For those who like more detail, when they hang out in threes, they become protons and neutrons). They are very happy when they are together, and, so they never have to be far from each other, there is an energy force that keeps them literally glued close together. This force is over one trillion trillion trillion times stronger than gravity. Since you just learned from $E = mc^2$ that energy is mass and mass is energy, then these gluon energy fields related to your quark threesomes also have a mass. As incredible as it may seem, it appears that this complex field composes the majority of your body mass! Remember the line "May the force be with you"? Well, you don't need to be a Jedi, because the force is already with you. In fact, physicists call this the "strong force."

I know that many of you are now thinking, "Dr. Bob, even though it is extremely enlightening and empowering to learn that the majority of the building blocks (the quarks) we are made of are maximally strong and teeming with force, it does seem that our quark trios are somewhat shy and are quite content staying within their 'shells.' Do we have a part of us that reflects the fun and exciting aspects of life? What about those electrons, Dr. Bob?"

No need to worry. Do you think that you would be created without perfect balance? No way! Let's talk about those electrons. Their personality is literally the opposite of those quark trio clusters, and they balance you out quite nicely. They are fun-loving, wild, excitable particles that are never shy to interact. Your electrons position themselves around a cluster of quark trios, where they oscillate and dance around at such a high speed that you really can't even pin them down to a certain point at any one time. They really do reflect your free-spirit side.

Recall how, on cold dry days when you rub your feet across the carpet and then lightly touch someone, it gives them a micro shock? Yes, those are fun-loving electrons at play. In fact, you could accurately say that your neighborhood is teeming with natural "electronicity" (to distinguish it from mankind-harnessed "unnatural" electricity) – another new word among many that you should consider adding to your vocabulary.

Thus, your neighborhood's natural state is a perfect balance of quarks and electrons in motion teeming with force and "electronicity"! In fact, motion is one of the signature features of our universe. Did you know that, to the best of our current knowledge, there is no matter that is completely motionless on Earth or in space, even in the depths of the known universe far away from any stars? Knowing how to align your thoughts, words, and actions with all of the natural universal energies and influences within this sea of motion will lay the foundation for your path to optimal wellness. Understanding your body's energetic nature is a critical step.

Time for answers…

Your individual quarks and electrons are perfect!

Your quarks and electrons "know" exactly how to interact and vibrate in perfect harmony to provide you with the capacity to have an extremely high level of quality of life. After all, they have had since the beginning of time to "bond" and work out all of their "differences!" And bond they do. Your quark families bond together by sharing their electrons with other quark families in your neighborhood to form everything from your DNA and cell membranes to your bony skeleton. Sounds like an active but peaceful neighborhood.

Yes, ideally, but what happens when "visitors" enter or pass through your neighborhood? This is what you have to know! You must learn which visitors are naturally good and sustaining, and which ones are intruders that aim to "gum up the works" or heat things up to the point that your electrons are literally jumping out of their shells and bonds are being broken. Since all energy is in motion, we can accurately call all of these "visitors" *energy-in-motion!*

The quantity of incoming energy-in-motion is staggering. As long as you consistently apply the knowledge that you are about to acquire, you can reduce the intruding energy to a level that your body can handle, which, in turn, creates space for healing energy. I've said it before and will say again: you have much more control over this than you may have been led to believe.

As you read on, please keep in mind that every page of text is presented in a specific and purposeful order. This is not a physics lesson. It is knowledge for your health and healing. It is time for you to update your vocabulary to reflect your true nature. You have one body…one vessel. Your body is energetically your closest "friend." If you choose to skim or gloss over any word, phrase, passage, or section, then you are caring less about your neighborhood. If you do not care about your neighborhood, your body will never be at ease. The truth is, "**Those who refuse to 'know' within… will go 'without'…**"

Your incredible epigenome

Before I walk you through the neighborhood, I want to make you aware of a major vibration within the body that has everybody "buzzing." It has been determined that there is a complex network of energy within your body that can control how your neighborhood DNA is expressed during your life ongoing. It has been named the epigenome, and it can play your DNA like a concert musician playing a finely tuned instrument. It is extremely sensitive to every bit of energy-in-motion that appears or resides in your neighborhood and it gets passed on to your future offspring!

An abundance of positive and natural energies and influences will permit good DNA vibrations to maintain body harmony and even reverse dis-ease. An abundance of negative and unnatural energetic influences will cause mass confusion within your neighborhood. This means that **regardless of the DNA "cards" that you have been dealt, it is your ability to apply the knowledge of what everything represents energetically that will mold your personal epigenome and allow you to realize your highest and best potential.** This jewel (or joule) of knowledge is incredibly important to keep in mind and carry forward.

Many have now acknowledged that it is time to replace the term disease with the more accurate "dis-ease." In other words, in virtually every state of chronic dis-ease, there always exists the *potential* to return your body to a state of ease. You just have to apply the keys!

Thus, the epigenome gives us a tangible evidence-based confirmation that the quality of your physical life does actually depend on knowing what represents a positive energetic influence and what represents a negative energetic influence, and then respectfully applying this knowledge, especially when it comes to your thoughts, words, and actions. The text will provide you with this knowledge.

Everything does matter!

CHAPTER TWO

VISITORS WITH ATTITUDE

We begin the journey by looking at four natural influences, all of which have "attitude." Their presence raises important points that you need to keep in mind as you travel through the text and through your life. By attitude, I do not mean to suggest that they are disruptive to your body. To the contrary, if they did not exist, it is likely that things would be quite different in and "around" your neighborhood. What I do mean by attitude is that these energies or influences either come and go as they please, are incredibly stubborn, or masquerade as one element when they would rather be another! Since they are present within your neighborhood every second of every day of your physical existence, wouldn't it be nice to know what they bring to your table, so to speak? I will now formally introduce you to these omnipresent guests.

Neutrinos

The ultimate passersby......or are they?

Let's begin with the ultimate passersby...the neutrinos. I know, it sounds like the name of a breakfast cereal. "Have you had your neutrinos today"? Yes, I know that's not funny. However, what is interesting is that you are actually "having" trillions and trillions of neutrinos for breakfast, lunch, dinner, and while you sleep! And they come in at least three quantum "flavors"! I'm not kidding...look it up!

These oscillating cosmic particles are hurtling through space at near the speed of light, but they pass through our bodies as if we didn't even exist. They leave virtually no calling cards, and, thus, it appears that your quarks and electrons do not even flinch at the "sight" of them. However, given the staggering number of neutrinos that visit your neighborhood every second of every day of your existence, is it possible that your body interacts with them in ways that we have yet to understand? Yes, and since you now know that every bit of mass is energy-in-motion, then at every point in time of your physical existence, these mysterious particles do contribute to your unique vibration. Thus, it is a fact that your neighborhood would be energetically different without them. In essence you would be a distinctly different "flavor"!

It is frequently the case that we do not respect and appreciate something natural until it becomes uncomfortably conspicuous by its absence. Clean fresh water, clean air, rainforests and other ecosystems are just a few obvious examples that are not a challenge to visualize and comprehend. In the same vein, you must never underestimate the significance of the "unseen" natural energies and influences. For example, I certainly do not have to explain what would happen if your natural supply of oxygen suddenly diminished. Given the fact that the sun is the source of most of your neutrinos, you will obviously not be experiencing a neutrino-free state in your lifetime. However, since our bodies have never existed in the absence of neutrinos, we do not know how important they are to us! In fact, if your body's natural "supply" of neutrinos were to suddenly plummet, this would mean that something catastrophic had happened to the sun. If something catastrophic happens to the sun…well, you do the math.

The point is, as you progress through the entire text and through your life ongoing, always have a healthy respect for all natural energies and influences, especially those that are meant to frequent your neighborhood. As you will learn, and as incredible as it may seem, **just beginning to cultivate a healthy mindset that acknowledges your body's energetic nature can, in itself, release barriers to wellness.** This is really important.

Gravity

"Hanging" around the neighborhood…

If you had to choose one natural phenomenon that is rock steady and, literally, brings you "down to Earth," there would be only one nominee. And the award goes to: *gravity*. We are taught about seventeenth century science relating to Sir Isaac Newton and a gravitational "force." We're often given the impression that it's old news in the history books and we know everything about it. Not even close!

The gravitational influence remains one of the unsolved mysteries of the physics world. Although we do know how to predict, with incredible accuracy, its effect on the movement of objects, planets, etc., we do not know how it does what it does. In other words, we can predict the time when a celestial event, such as a solar eclipse, will occur thirty years from now, but physicists are still attempting to find a particle that can explain the "attractiveness" of gravitation. They have even reserved the term "graviton" to name this particle if they ever find it.

Our bodies experience gravitation as a subtle, or not-so-subtle, nudge to move closer to everything around us. You read earlier that gravitational "attractiveness" is relatively weak when compared to forces such as those that keep you glued together. However, although you may not consciously perceive the attraction towards every object in every direction, *your body does.* The major gravitational effect that we are all familiar with is, of course, the one that keeps our feet on the surface of Mother Earth.

The effect of gravitation has always been and will always be hanging around your neighborhood…no matter where or how far you travel. In fact, the astronauts' bodies that seem to be "floating" in an orbiting spacecraft still experience roughly 90% of the gravitational effect that we experience on Earth's surface. Did you know that the astronauts are not floating at all…they are actually in free-fall due to…Earth's gravitational influence!

What if I told you that you could "blame" your weight on gravity? Before you jump on the anti-gravity bandwagon, let me explain. Remember who you are…the **m** in the $E = mc^2$, and **m** does not stand for weight. It is mass, which you now know is the total amount of stuff, or matter, that you are made of…your perfect neighborhood quarks, electrons, and forces. Your mass may weigh 150 pounds on Earth, but you would also weigh 25 pounds on the moon and 57 pounds on Mars.

Thus, gravity is responsible for the number we call weight, and as long as we continue to live on the surface of this planet, it does give us a reference point to determine our mass at any particular moment. However, it does not cause us to become more "mass-ive." That, of course, occurs when we retain more energy than our body releases.

So, can gravity stress us in? No, it cannot. Gravitation is an ever-present universal influence on your neighborhood, that is nontoxic! However, if you allow your body's neighborhood to stagnate and become congested, or you choose to engage in aggressive, high impact activities, you will change the status quo between your body and gravity, and sooner or later there will be consequences.

Let's examine how this works:

The health impact on your body specifically related to gravity is more complex than you may realize. From now on, **refer to gravity as the "tug of vitality"** as it works with your body to strengthen your neighborhood. Yes, the integrity of your musculoskeletal system depends on your purposeful movement within the sea of gravity. Also, the healthy flow of your neighborhood's superhighways, tributaries, and branches that you know as your lymphatic and circulatory systems is dependent on a precise body-gravity relationship.

Here are the three rules of engagement for gravity to work in harmony with you:

1) **Naturally easing your body to a mass that is most optimal with gravity is critical to your longevity.** As long as you treat your neighborhood with respect, your genome and epigenome will ensure that your physical structure is just the right mass to work in harmony with the Earth's gravitational field. Since at least a billion people in the world are over-mass, it is clear that we have major issues to address, individually and collectively. So, how do you know what your optimal mass is and how do you achieve this goal?

Historically, we have used the term "overweight" to describe a person who is over-mass. People pick a target "weight" from a chart of questionable validity, then use an incomplete set of keys and struggle to reach that goal before yo-yoing back up again. More recently, many use a body-mass index as a guide. (Note that it is not called a body-weight index.) However, even though this terminology is more accurate, most people who are over-mass still struggle to maintain an optimal mass due to their incomplete knowledge of what obesity represents energetically.

The bottom line: As long as you consistently apply all the keys presented within the text, your body will repay you in kind by easing to your optimal mass, which is an essential key to your physical longevity!

2) It is a myth that you must support any region of your neighborhood beyond its natural structural integrity. Here is an example that has relevance to a high profile issue in health today. Because serious breast dis-ease is so prevalent and one of the most devastating manifestations of being stressed in, it has even been debated as to whether or not breast support garments (e.g., brassieres) cause breast dis-ease. The more accurate question is, "Does a breast support garment alter the status quo between the body and the gravitational field, *potentially* contributing to the development of serious breast dis-ease?" The answer is absolutely yes! Energetically, by resisting gravity in this manner, you are changing it from a "tug of vitality" to a "tug of war."

In addition, it is a physiological fact that you can alter the natural flow of your neighborhood's highways (the lymphatics and blood vessels) to and from the breasts, or any other area of the body, by the pressure applied by a support garment. Thus, anything that resists gravity's beneficial "tug" or restricts flow, by definition, stresses you in. You would be wise to intelligently and respectfully limit the time bound by any restrictive garments.

I should mention that another "support device" which alters your status quo with gravity is the shoe. More podiatric, orthopedic, and even circulatory dis-ease can be attributed to wearing shoes than you can imagine. Since most of your daily routines "require" you to navigate terrain that is not foot-friendly, you obviously cannot just abandon the shoe. However, whenever appropriate and possible, remove your shoes and give your skeleton and muscles more time to equilibrate with natural gravity! In fact, when appropriate, please allow daily time for your bare feet to directly contact Mother Earth. Those free-spirit electrons at play again. Your body will love you for it.

3) The third rule of engagement has to do with purposeful motion within the sea of gravity. In other words…exercise. This optimizes the "tug of vitality" and the healthy flow of your neighborhood's highways! An intelligent and naturally impacting aerobic routine using your legs and arms will allow gravity to work at its best for you. Your bones will be stronger and you will reap many other proven benefits, including **improved brain function!**

Then, once your body is warmed up and in the flow from your natural exercise, do not forget about simple stretching. As you carefully stretch, allow your body to guide you to a "feel good" place. This is a good spot to "hang out." If your body sends you a symptom of pain, that is guidance to ease away for the moment.

Please be aware that playing in a sporting event is not equivalent to exercise. Exercise is restorative, maintaining, and in-sync with gravity. Given the incidence of injury and body dis-ease directly related to sporting event participation, it is clear that virtually all athletics take the body out of alignment with gravity in some way. Knee, ankle, and shoulder injuries are among the most common.

There is another consequence of misalignment with gravity that, until recently, parents have been afraid to "look straight in the eye." That is, the risk of brain dis-ease caused by the use of the head within the guidelines of certain sports, especially soccer and gridiron football. The head was never meant to be a backboard. Thus, there is no such thing as purposeful heading, helmet or no helmet. As a parent, you have an obligation to share this knowledge with your child.

I know that there are those who, due to neuro/musculoskeletal injury or degenerative neuro/musculoskeletal dis-ease, cannot freely engage the "tug of vitality." If you can engage carefully and to the best of your ability and apply all of the other keys of knowledge presented in the text, you have the potential to experience a sense of ease that you may have not thought possible.

Jewels (joules) to keep in mind:

Remind yourself that gravitation is no longer relegated to a question on a physics test. It is a neighborhood influence that has always been and will always be tugging at your body strings. It is ultra-esoteric and may have properties beyond our current knowledge. Start to refer to yourself in terms of mass. The term "body-mass index" is already in use…not "body-weight index." If you choose to step on a scale, say you **gained mass** or **released mass**. This is more accurate and an acknowledgment that you are current with the new paradigm. Why the term "released"? Because **mass cannot be lost in the universe. It becomes energy in a different space.** It is profoundly important to actively engage the gravitational field. As you exercise intelligently, mindfully acknowledge that your greatest ally of structural function and integrity is the "tug of vitality." After all, healthy exercise = purposeful motion within the sea of gravity = direct or indirect benefit to every area of your neighborhood, including improved brain function. Visualize your neighborhood within to motivate yourself to work with gravity following the three laws of engagement. Your body will love you for it!

Potassium-40 and Carbon-14

Renegade troops? ...or natural ally?

If you remember the famous story of Paul Revere, you recall that he set up a system where one lit lantern would warn of dangerous troops from the land and two lanterns danger from the sea. If there could be a warning cry for the body, it might be:

40 if by land, 14 if by C

However, in this case, your neighborhood can stand at ease…

For as long as the Earth has existed, there have been elements (metals, gases, etc.) that are just not content to stay what they are. For example, a small percentage of potassium atoms would rather be argon or calcium! They are known as K-40. Their transformation occurs as the result of a single quark changing its vibration! (I never said that your quarks didn't have a sense of humor.) Since potassium is abundant in our soil and food and we cannot survive without it, some of this potassium is always present within our bodies.

Another transformer that we find in the neighborhood is called Carbon-14. We call this "14 if by C," because this element is not actually produced in the sea. Energy-in-motion from the "big sea" – the Cosmos – triggers the production of this carbon naturally in our atmosphere. These carbons would rather be nitrogens. They enter our bodies through almost everything we ingest. Since these transformers are present within your body every second of every day of your physical life, they also contribute to your natural vibratory flavor.

However, as these elements transform themselves within your body, bits of energy-in-motion are released which can be irritating to other nearby residents of your neighborhood. This would appear to be concerning since carbon-14's are also naturally found within the structure of your DNA. So, what gives? Are they natural allies or are they party crashers?

As always, we must not overlook the perfect order and good purpose that nature seems always to provide. Did you know that your body is equipped with mechanisms to repair energetic micro-trauma that occurs within your neighborhood? Yes, you have a very high level repair team within you. Is it possible, then, that your naturally positioned K-40's and C-14's are integrally related to the creation and ongoing efficiency of your complex and vital DNA repair team? Yes, and you can be sure that they exist in harmony after all this time. Thus, the relationship between these residents and your body's DNA repair mechanism must be considered a natural status quo within your neighborhood, and thus, by definition, naturally occurring C-14's and K-40's are not intruders and do not stress you in. Think of these natural transformers as keeping your body's repair team alert and primed for action!

So, it's all okay? Unfortunately not, because above-ground nuclear testing decades ago dramatically increased the amount of carbon-14 in the atmosphere. Thus, the status quo was changed. It is well documented that the increased carbon-14 has entered our bodies even long after the nuclear testing was stopped. Thus, the increased degree of atomic (pun intended) micro-trauma to the body caused by these mankind-released C-14's is real, and, by definition, they have added to the *cumulative stress-in effect* on your neighborhood, whether directly or through inherited DNA alterations. This is only a tip of the iceberg of the many mankind-generated threats to your DNA, as you will learn.

Joules to keep in mind:

Aside from the obvious fact that mankind-generated nuclear explosions stress in everybody on the planet and absolutely have no place within the natural fabric, there is an intriguing question regarding your body's transformers that may come to mind. That is, "Is there such a thing as 'good' stress and, if so, could our naturally positioned potassium-40's and carbon-14's be classified as a type of 'good' stress?" The answer is no, and no. **There is no good stress!** From the definition of stress you now know that stress involves a disruption of the *harmony* of your natural neighborhood processes. As you learned, your naturally positioned neighborhood potassium-40's and carbon-14's are already within the natural harmony. They have always been and will always be ingredients that contribute to your natural vibration.

There are still those who would like you to believe that there is "good" stress. They equate life's challenges with stress. This is false. If they mean to say that life's emotional challenges can teach us lessons that can prepare us for our lives ongoing, then we have something to talk about. As you will learn, **challenges are not equivalent to stress!**

Radon: a breath of "stress" air?

Before we move on, there is a fifth visitor with attitude, radon, another transformer from the earth, that you must be made aware of.

What comes to mind when you hear the word "uranium"? Nuclear weapons…radioactive decay…espionage…fear? Well, don't panic, but there is uranium in the soil under your feet just about everywhere on the planet, and, yes, it is undergoing radioactive decay. If it were willing to stay in the soil we would not be having this discussion. But, you guessed it: uranium is another atom that is just not content with continuing on as just uranium. In fact, it desires to become a non-radioactive form of lead. It is such a massive atom that it must reinvent itself many times before reaching its goal. It is truly one of nature's premier transformers.

One of its forms happens to be a gas called radon, which filters up through the soil and into the air. It naturally hovers near the ground, gets moved around by air currents and gets dispersed fairly easily. Unfortunately, mankind again has changed the status quo of nature. With our desire to create more living space – such as basements – and our ability to design our dwellings to be more "hermetically" sealed to "protect" us from the elements, we have given radon space to become trapped and to concentrate within a confined area, where our bodies are then exposed to levels beyond that which nature intended.

What you have to know is that exposure to radon at levels above that which nature intended is considered to be the major factor for the development of lung cancer in people who ***do not*** smoke! How devastating would it be if, despite an organic and holistically oriented lifestyle, you were diagnosed with lung cancer, which causes more deaths per year than any other cancer?

Thus, have your dwelling and workplace tested for radon gas, especially if you have a basement or spend time in rooms or dwellings that are below the ground level. Do not be led into a false sense of security by anyone who says you don't have to test because you live in a low radon area or that your neighbor's house tested safe. Two houses next door to each other can have dramatically different levels. Just do it. It could literally save you from manifesting life threatening dis-ease.

A real "smoking gun"...

As radon rises out of the soil on tobacco farms, the radioactive particles that form like to stick to the furry leaves of the tobacco plants. When a person lights a cigarette, these particles become airborne again. Thus, as one smokes or you breathe in second-hand smoke, you are becoming more radioactive! In fact, it has been estimated that smoking, even modestly, can be the equivalent of exposing your lungs to dozens of x-rays per year. Your body also has to deal with the airborne particles that move to your bloodstream, which may be contributing to the development of other dis-ease as well. What about third-hand smoke? Yes, the residue of burned tobacco smoke even on clothes and other surfaces can stress you in. In addition, as your epigenome is exposed to your tobacco habit, the negative influence can be potentially passed on to your future children and their descendants!

Thus, as a smoker, you are not only disrespecting your own neighborhood, but you may also be passing on the consequences of your habit to undermine the health of your future offspring! Every one of you who smokes tobacco is, at least to some degree, self-medicating symptoms of internalized emotional stress energy. You all know the truth of that statement. Later in the text, you will learn how to manage, recycle, and release these energies, and you will be able to move away from the smoking habit more easily! Your body, and your children, will love you for it.

Additional joules:

For those who have previously heard of radon, you know that radon is generally thought of as something to fear, and to blame if one suspects that it was linked to their body dis-ease. It's time to set the record straight. As you will learn, fear and blame, in themselves, are hindrances to wellness. Fearing and blaming any natural element cultivates a mindset that is misaligned with nature and clouds your view of how to achieve optimal balance within the natural fabric. For example, would you blame gravity if you were to fall and sprain your ankle? Can you blame the sun for a burn if you overexposed yourself to its direct rays? Can we really blame radon if we are not thoughtful or careful enough to respect its boundaries? The point is, **natural elements are not here to stress us in.** It is our lack of knowledge about them or our lack of respect for their natural boundaries that can lead to negative consequences. As you acquire a solid foundation of knowledge and adjust your mindset accordingly, it is guaranteed that your body will respond in kind.

CHAPTER THREE

THE SILENCE OF THE WAVES

Silent and invisible waves are engaging and interacting with your body all of the time. Many of you are being blind-sided along your path to optimal health, as you have not been given a proper foundation of knowledge regarding the most common spectrum of these waves. It's time for you to "see" what's really going on in this vast "sea".

A wave is produced when something moves or vibrates. We all are familiar with waves we can see and hear. Ocean waves would be an obvious example. If movement occurs anywhere from the ocean floor to the surface of the ocean, a wave is generated. If you drop a pebble in the water you see the waves rippling out in all directions.

We also take sound waves for granted. Molecules in the air are vibrated to cause their own ripple effect until this "ripple" reaches your eardrum and causes it to vibrate. Did you know that in space, outside of the Earth's atmosphere, there are not enough molecules of gas to sustain a ripple of any significant magnitude to vibrate our eardrums enough to make sound? Thus, if you could set off fireworks while in space, the visual display would be spectacular but you would not hear a sound! As you know, sound waves can stress you in if you allow yourself continuous or even intermittent exposure to very loud sounds. Don't take this lightly, and be sure to teach your children well in this regard, as any disrespect that you show to your neighborhood's auditory processors will, later in life, make it more difficult for your body to accurately process the incoming energy when engaged by another person or situation. In addition, sound does not have to be loud to stress you in! I will discuss the dissonance of noise later in the text.

What about the "silent" waves that you cannot see or hear? Many of these are the subject of great controversy, as you will soon learn. These waves are called *electromagnetic waves* and we will discuss them in terms of *tiny packets of energy called photons.* They are generated by movement and vibrations at a quantum level and they want to get where they are going…and fast. They move naturally at approximately 300,000,000 meters per second.

POP QUIZ: How many of the following waves did we, as humans, introduce first?

	Light
Radio	Ultraviolet
Micro	X-Ray
Infrared	Gamma

ANSWER: Zero.

The universe has held the patent on these since the beginning of time. Mankind has exploited the electron and even the quark in an attempt to harness the power of the universe with very mixed results. One could argue that all of mankind's attempts have been less than optimal reproductions that have fallen short of the mark. Actually, there is no argument…it is a fact.

These seven waves are found in abundance within our universe. Earth's atmosphere filters or blocks them to varying degrees, allowing just the right amount of wave energy to reach the surface of the Earth, where our bodies exist in harmony with them. Once again, however, mankind altered the status quo when we found our own ways to generate these waves, thus over-exposing our bodies and stressing us in.

These waves can all be described as packets of energy called, as you read earlier, photons. They differ only in how much energetic punch they can deliver when something (like your body) gets in their way. To give you an idea of how vast the spectrum of energy is, imagine you are wading in the shallow water at the beach and you are impacted by one wave per hour. Let's say this wave represents an FM radio photon wave. In comparison, a medical x-ray photon wave would be equivalent to you being impacted by over one billion waves per hour! This is clearly intolerable and would leave at least some scars. Does this mean that the FM radio frequency wave is safe? No it does not! The misconception that these lower energy waves of technology, including cellular phone waves, do not stress us in has been one of the great tragedies of the modern era. Let's take a look at these "not so silent" waves.

Meet the Photons...

Let there be light!

Illuminating (rainbow) waves

For most of mankind's recorded history, people have equated light with the capacity of the sun to illuminate the surroundings. Of course, fire (via candle, torch, etc.) was used to penetrate the darkness. In the last 150 years we have added the electric bulb to the mix. The word "light" has been of intrinsic significance in both the works of physicists and in the realm of spiritual script. Nature's illumination is most beautiful and humbling as we experience the sun, lightning, and the northern lights (aurora), to name the most obvious. Only the precise blend of rainbow photons that we know as sunlight can keep us healthy and vibrant. Let's give the word "light" the respect it deserves and reserve it for referring to natural universal illumination, the highest and the best being from the illuminating-rainbow spectrum of photons from the sun.

The blend of photons from the electric bulb has always been and will always be inferior. The bulb's generic brand is faux (meaning 'fake' and pronounced exactly like *pho*-) and always stresses you in. From now on, if you think of the bulb as producing a "fauxton" blend of illumination, you will be more likely to take action to reduce your time spent under "the bulb."

Our sun has been the Earth's source of illuminating waves forever. Whether you believe in a purely scientific view of the big bang, spiritual scripture's description of the emergence of "light", or both, illuminating waves are the most critical to our lives. Did you know that these photon waves are so important that, to the best of our knowledge, the sun "holds on" to every one of them for thousands of years before releasing them to us! This certainly places the meaning of the word "patience" in a whole new light, wouldn't you say?

Our bodies are perfectly adapted to the exact spectrum of illuminating waves the sun sends out consistently. In fact, when these waves hit the back of our eye, signals are also sent to the ultimate balancing organ of our body, the hypothalamus, which in turn communicates to the area – the pineal gland – that regulates melatonin production.

Thus, a healthy biological clock and its ability to reset require the sun's "brand" of illuminating waves. It is well known that many who are inadequately exposed to these "sunny" waves are not at ease. Those of you who live in perpetually cloudy locations or who are otherwise "sun-deprived" know the truth of this.

As we have discussed, mankind's attempt to copy the sun resulted in the electric bulb. Working all day and spending evenings bathed in these sun impostors has become the standard of society. It stresses you in more than you may know!

What can you do?

There are some newer bulbs that emit illuminating waves that are closer to the sun's brand. You should do your research and consider replacing your older bulbs. You should encourage your employers to do the same if you spend several hours a day under the fauxton blend of the bulb. Since the standard incandescent bulbs actually use more energy to heat the glass bulb than to provide illumination, there has been a movement to require the use of more "energy-efficient" compact fluorescent bulbs whenever possible. However, all bulbs present their own risks.

One potential problem is that the "more efficient" fluorescent bulbs contain mercury, which is actually a rare natural element that, through mining, has been displaced from its safe haven below the surface of the Earth. Thus, if the bulb should break, you could be exposed to this displaced mercury and become stressed-in. Handle these bulbs with care and be sure to dispose of them according to environmentally friendly guidelines. Also, fluorescents can produce a greater electromagnetic field of undesirable energy that is of no benefit to your neighborhood. This "field of fluorescents" could actually be another emerging barrier to wellness.

The bottom line is that all bulbs will stress you in to some extent and have the potential to contribute to more serious body dis-ease. Do your best to find ways to improve access to sunlight within your house. For example, installing skylights, larger windows, or removing obstructions to sunlight, to name a few. Those who work in offices that are bright enough during the day to obviate the need for turning on the lights can be expected to have better focus, experience less fatigue, and be more at ease! In addition, be aware that working during the night and sleeping during the day goes against your natural daily biological clock. This is not optimal and always stresses you in.

As easy as A, B, C *and D?*

Ultraviolet waves

Birds see it. Bees see it. I'm not sure if educated fleas see it. I am not referring to a Cole Porter song. I'm referring to *ultraviolet* (UV) waves that are not illuminating for humans but your body certainly needs them. These waves are most well known for their tanning ability. They are more energetic waves than light waves.

The sun has three brands – A, B, and C. Since many of you have become obsessed with the appearance of the largest component of your neighborhood – your skin – ultraviolet waves have been a high profile topic of controversy for many years. Brand A is always being blamed and held responsible for accelerating your skin's aging process as it travels beneath the surface to your tissues and elastic components of your skin. Brand B is more energetic and has become feared for its potential to cause burns. Highly energetic Brand C, for good reason, has been delegated to stay out of reach in the Cosmos, and fortunately is blocked from reaching Earth's surface through the work of our good friends oxygen and ozone.

Ultraviolet waves have also taken the brunt of the blame when it comes to certain eye conditions such as cataracts. As always, it will be in your best interest to stop blaming or fearing natural energies and begin to acquire knowledge regarding what their good purpose may be. **The natural beauty of your skin and the integrity of your eye health are much more dependent on the beauty of your mind and avoidance of unnatural influences, such as cigarette smoke, alcohol, and poor dietary choices!**

So, what are these waves really good for? A lot, as it turns out. Once again, the universe had planned ahead. For starters, because a variety of birds, bees, bats and fish use ultraviolet waves to find food, prey, and mates, without these waves ecosystems would be out of balance and distinctly different from what we see today. For example, our flying friends use ultraviolet to locate and pollinate many flowers. Also, to protect their internal integrity from ultraviolet, fruits actually manufacture their own "sunscreens," some of which just so happen to be the healthy pigments and antioxidants that we require! Our healthy food choices would be very limited if our atmosphere did not allow the passage of ultraviolet waves.

Our atmosphere does not allow free passage of the brand B waves, but it does let just enough pass through for a very good reason. UVB waves actually transform a form of cholesterol in your skin to a vitally important factor that is commonly referred to as Vitamin D. Interestingly, to be most accurate, vitamin D is not a vitamin at all…it is actually a hormone! Please remember this…it is a very important distinction. Think about it…a hormone produced with the sun as a catalyst! You can be sure that the "Sun hormone" is much more important than we know. It is essential for proper bone metabolism and in many other ways. There are relatively few natural food sources with an abundance of vitamin D. Thus, instead of focusing on the possibility that UV burns, always remember that UVB = Vitamin D…the Sun hormone.

What you need to know about exposure to UV

The consequences of misaligning your body with the sun's UV through *overexposure* (i.e., burns) can leave your skin cells more vulnerable to dis-ease. On the other hand, the consequences of misaligning your body with the sun's UV through *underexposure* (i.e., vitamin D deficiency) can leave your *entire body* more vulnerable to dis-ease! Thus, the mindset that has prevailed over the last half century that we must pour on the sunscreen to "protect" us from the sun's waves has been a healthcare disaster. We have also become a society obsessed with sunglasses. Please do not use sunscreen or wear sunglasses all of the time, unless you have an exceptionally rare extenuating medical circumstance that would guide you otherwise. In fact, the strategic use of sunglasses or sunscreen should be considered only under specific conditions, such as exceptionally bright locations or if one anticipates a prolonged exposure risk.

All exposure to ultraviolet will stimulate release of pre-packaged pigment and production of new pigment in the skin at least to some degree (tanning). This occurs naturally as we strive to optimize our level of "Sunny D." The pertinent question is, how much exposure is naturally safe? The line between just enough UV to generate maximal Sun hormone and to avoid burns is not well demarcated and varies from individual to individual.

In essence, you have your individual status quo that you need to determine to the best of your ability.

So, how do we begin to respectfully engage the sun's UV waves? In all cases, opt to the cautious side to start. Begin by setting aside as little as ten minutes per day, three to four days per week, to soak up the sun's UV without any sunscreen, preferably when the sun is highest in the sky. Yes, the greatest access to the sun's UVB comes at midday, especially if you live at the higher latitudes. Expose as much of your body surface as is appropriate and respectful for the venue. As long as you are careful not to burn, you can work your minutes up to twenty, and even moderately beyond. Again, the amount of time varies from person to person and it will take some trial and error to get the entire routine to the level that's optimal for you. If your skin is more generously pigmented, you will need more time to soak up the sun's UV. Be aware that even the youngest of children require these sunny waves also, but take "baby" steps, as you must avoid burns!

If you do anticipate a situation where the strategic use of sunscreen appears warranted, be sure to research sunscreens and blocks for the safest ingredients and the waves you want to block. Everything that you apply to your skin can potentially be absorbed and stress you in, so do your homework as to the safety of the ingredients.

Please note that UVA may travel through glass but UVB has difficulty. Thus avoid direct sun through glass at all times. They say that people who live in glass houses shouldn't throw stones…but please feel free to open your windows once and a while to allow the sun to provide you with the catalyst to produce your Sun hormone!

You will be hearing much more about your vitamin D/Sun hormone, as it is one of the hot topics in healing and health at the moment. Its effect on your immune system is especially complex. Is it possible that in the fall and winter months, when most of us are covered up and sun-deprived, you are more susceptible to cold and flu specifically because your sunny-D levels drop? This is a most plausible hypothesis. In addition, sunny-D may also attenuate many other states of dis-ease, from auto-immune to cancer. Do your research and stay very in tune to the evolving guidelines for testing your D levels and how to support these levels in times when you are truly sun-deprived.

Also, if you are a woman who expects to be pregnant in the not so distant future or you are presently pregnant, please keep in mind that you have two bodies to supply with the Sun hormone. It is vitally important that you do not allow yourself to become Sun hormone-deprived, as an adequate supply of Sun hormone to the child in your womb is critical in preparation for the child's early months of life outside your womb. This is really important! In case you are wondering, your body naturally ensures that you will not produce "too much" vitamin D from exposure to sunny waves alone.

Additional joules for thought:

Is it possible that movement within the sea of gravity as you are exposed to the sun's UV waves could be even more optimal for you? In other words, if you are going to be spending time in the sun, then instead of just sunbathing, could it be more optimal if you walk, garden or at least move around in some manner as your body is exposed to your dose of the sun's UV? Yes, and this is not surprising, as you have chosen to engage two natural universal energies simultaneously. Your body will love you for it!

Waves of convenience...risky business

Radio, micro, cell phones, and others

The twentieth century could certainly be described as the time in history when we lost our healthy respect for nature and became smug about our ability to harness its power. We have become a society where the quest for convenience and the quantity of possessions has progressed with little regard for the possible consequences. We have seen the negative health effects of processing foods for mass production and convenience. We will shortly discuss one of the many problems related to fossil fuels which resulted from our love affair with gasoline-powered machines and the need for speed. These are just two examples where the cat is already out of the bag. There exists another major issue in the form of mankind-generated wave pollution that society, again, seems to have swept under the rug.

Radio waves and microwaves are abundant throughout the universe. In fact, the entire universe is bathed in a primordial soup of microwaves. Isn't it ironic that we now use mankind-harnessed microwaves to unnaturally heat our own soup? Yes, the consumption of microwave-heated food will stress you in. On a more profound note, years before the microwave oven, we found a way to generate types of waves that could carry information such as audio (to the radio) and video (to the television). Since then, our appetite for instant access to audio-visual stimuli has escalated to where we believe that we cannot live prosperous and gratifying lives without a 24/7 connection to our world through advanced technology in this realm, including cellular phones. Notable examples include waves to AM/FM radio, television, cellular phones, our computers via wireless routers, and even garage doors and car door locks via remote control. Thus, our environment is saturated with these mankind-generated photon waves.

The ongoing controversy and debate has been whether or not these waves cause harm to our bodies. Wrong question...wrong debate. The more accurate question is, do these waves stress you in, with the potential to contribute to the development of serious body dis-ease? With your new knowledge of energy-in-motion, you can see that the answer clearly must be yes.

Here's why: There are few, if any, elements in the universe that our bodies are virtually transparent to. As we have discussed, the neutrino may be one of them, but even that is not a certainty. On the other hand, it is a fact that your body can *feel* all waves, including these lower energy audio-visual waves. It may be at an extremely subtle and esoteric level, but nevertheless your neighborhood is aware of them. Thus, when any photon wave enters your neighborhood, vibrations change slightly and your body must work to recalibrate this vibration. The effect of these bits of disruptive energy could potentially weaken certain body systems, such as our complex immune system, in ways that we have yet to understand. They could also potentially agitate the highly sensitive structures deep within our brain. If an abundance of these waves are focused close to your body in a specific location, as could happen from a cell phone pressed against your head, more unwanted energy will be released from nearby cells internally as your body tries to keep balance, and, thus, the potential exists for these waves alone to lead to more serious dis-ease.

What you can do...

Mankind-generated wave pollution is a real threat to your body. It is an insidious invisible cloud that may be slowly eroding our state of natural health. As more wireless devices send increased quantities of these waves towards your neighborhood at breakneck speed, your body will have to devote more of its resources to maintaining your neighborhood within. Do not hold your breath waiting for some "official" agency to say, "Oops, we should have warned you sooner," about the possible hazards.

Since we do not know whether the stress-in effect of these waves is additive or multiplies the stress-in effects from all other sources combined, it would be best for you to take inventory of the quantity of your own individual exposure to these waves (any wireless devices or proximity to commercial transmitters, etc.). Research and do what you can to limit your exposure. Unless you require an active wireless source for emergency reasons, then please turn your wireless boxes and gadgets off at night while you are asleep.

Wireless waves of convenience are not likely to be pulled from society anytime soon, so just being aware that they do stress you in and that they do pose a threat is a good start. Since more people will now be aware of this potential threat, you should know that if you allow cell phone towers, masts, or other wireless tower stations within the vicinity of your home, school, or business, the desirability of your location will be negatively impacted.

Waves that really hurt...

Gamma and X

These waves cause serious *mass confusion* within your body. These waves are often called rays, which does drive home the point that they can penetrate deeply and destructively. They cause your electrons to jump out of their shells and break your bonds to a point where your cells may never be able to fully recover. Fortunately, our atmosphere does a great job of denying space gammas and X's entry to the surface of the Earth.

However, mankind has found a way to harness Earth gammas and X's to diagnose and treat stressed-in areas within our bodies. You are familiar with x-rays and C-T (a.k.a. CAT) scans, both in the realm of X. You may have heard of PET scans, which measure gamma waves from the radioactive material that is injected directly into one's neighborhood. Although the quantity of time one is exposed to these diagnostic tests is "relatively" low, they always disrupt your neighborhood and thus always stress you in.

When used to treat, a much more energetic dose of these waves is aimed at an already stressed-in area of the body – the deeply stressed-in cells known as cancer. These gammas and X's may well destroy the stressed-in cells, but they do not always spare the surrounding natural cells – certainly a difficult situation. Of course, we have misused the energy of the quark to the nth degree since we built and used nuclear weapons, which released deadly amounts of various waves that really hurt…

What you have to know about gamma rays and x-rays

The X-waves of C-T scans alone could leave your cells vulnerable to becoming deeply stressed-in, even long after the exposure. Thus, we have another confirmation that you must carefully weigh the risks versus benefits of X or gamma testing, especially where a child is concerned. Only agree to an x-ray or scan if it is absolutely necessary. Since all x-rays stress you in, there is no such thing as a routine x-ray or scan! For example, if you have a preventive care physical exam and the practitioner says a chest x-ray is part of the routine solely based on "age" or for "completeness," you should certainly request specific information that supports the benefit versus the risk of this test.

What about spinal x-rays? There are many of you who agree to a complete set of spine x-rays without considering the risk versus benefit. If your practitioner does not have a high level of suspicion that you have a vertebral fracture or imminently threatening bone disease, please ask questions before you allow x-rays into your neighborhood. For those of you with chronic symptoms of back pain, did you know that your body may respond more favorably to an adjustment of your mindset than it would to a lifetime of spinal adjustments?

Another high profile issue is mammography. Conventional mammograms, by definition, stress you in. The debate over the risk/benefit ratio of this procedure continues to rage on. There has been a natural way to image breast tissue for several years but it is only now gaining traction in the conventional world. It is called thermography and uses our own natural body waves in the realm of infrared to detect areas of concern. We will discuss infrared waves shortly.

You should know that air travel always stresses you in. Excess cosmic rays gain access to your neighborhood and force your body's DNA repair team to work that much harder. Will frequent air travel lead to obvious dis-ease? It may or may not...but that is not the question. The point is that it adds to the collective energies that stress you in, and thus has the potential to contribute to more serious dis-ease. It's another energy that your DNA has to deal with.

Vitally important joules:

If you effectively apply all of the knowledge presented within the text, it is certain that you and your children will have significantly less chance of ever needing diagnostic tests that involve gammas or X's, and less chance of ever having to undergo high energy X or gamma procedures. Your body will love you for it!

They're not imaginary,
and they are very unnerving...

ELF fields

Electricity is the most commonly known product of humanity's ability to harness the power of the excitable electron. As you know, power lines electrify our dwellings so that we can "plug in" and "light up." These lines and transformers produce extremely low frequency (ELF) waves that are even less energetic than the radio waves, but as you now know, they still invade our neighborhood space. Because power lines are so abundant and relatively close to the ground, many of you have been living within the electromagnetic field produced by these lines. As with the other "waves of convenience," there has also been considerable debate as to the health effects of living within the boundaries of these fields or working in the proximity of power lines. This debate will go on and on, but again, these waves and fields absolutely stress you in and have the potential to contribute to to more serious dis-ease.

Not unexpectedly, the Earth appears to have its own ELF signature. This is natural and may well serve to compliment our own natural vibes. Disturbingly, the frequency generated by electric power lines is near the upper range of your own brainwaves. In addition to being present at times of greatest awareness, these brainwaves may also be linked with your ability to form and retrieve memory!

Consider the possible implications. **Could these mankind-generated electromagnetic fields be distorting your memories of your ongoing life experiences as well as interfering with your brain's ability to promote restful sleep?** Given the fact that two of the most high profile issues in healthcare today involve the significance of subtle memory disturbances as well as the epidemic of sleep disorders, I would say that you should take notice. Could there be a link between electromagnetic fields and dementia? Serious stuff, wouldn't you say? Talk about mass confusion along your life's path...

What you can do…

You can actually purchase a field detector that can help you to identify the "stress energy" spots in your dwellings and your surroundings. Identifying these spots can tip you off to areas within your walls that may need attention. It certainly would be helpful to know if the head of your bed is next to a "hot" spot behind the wall, for example. Your brain certainly does not need to deal with that while you are sleeping. If you are looking at an office to rent, bring along your detector, especially if you work in the healing arts or use devices sensitive to energy fields. Many of you are working in the midst of these disruptive fields. Also, weigh the benefits against the potential risks if you are considering buying a home directly adjacent to a power line or transformer.

Many of you spend significant time in your automobile. Where there are live batteries and wires, there are fields when the ignition is engaged. In traditional vehicles the field would be greatest closer to the front end. That means you, the driver, may be bathed in a significant field of unwanted energy. Some hybrids have a battery mid-car, thus the back seat may be a concern. Thus, in addition to the fact that highway exhaust fumes produce "stress-air," you now have another reason to minimize your time in the car.

Also, be aware that electric appliances, when operating, will generate a very high field close to the appliance itself. This includes hairdryers, shavers, fans, toasters, and clock radios, among others. Do you really need all of these appliances? It is in your best interest to reduce your time spent in proximity to mankind-generated electric currents. Your body will love you for it!

We're having a "heat wave"...

Infrared waves

From our lesson on motion, we know that no object is energetically frozen in its tracks, and thus, the excitable electrons of every object continue to vibrate, jump around, and interact. What is the one wave we can count on to confirm that everything on Earth has a "pulse," so to speak? That would be the infrared wave. No matter how stone cold an object looks, there are still IR waves that can potentially be emitted. For example, an ice cube radiates IR even though we don't perceive it as such. We can "see" this energy using infrared detectors, such as those used by law enforcement personnel and astrophysicists. We can feel these waves as heat. Did you know that ear thermometers display your temperature based on the amount of IR emitted from your eardrum?

Also, as was discussed in the previous section, we are now recognizing the validity of safely measuring our infrared signature to detect areas of dis-ease. Thermography is being looked at as a promising alternative to mammography.

Planet Earth has its own unique infrared signal, which is enhanced by the illuminating (rainbow) waves of the sun. If our atmosphere allowed all of these infrared waves to radiate out into space, we would quickly move into an ice age. (The average surface temperature of the entire planet would plummet.) Fortunately, nature comes through again, as water vapor in the air and other gases grab these waves and create a warming blanket for the Earth.

One of these gases is CO^2 (carbon dioxide) which, as you know, has received worldwide attention in recent years. Burning of fossil fuels (motor vehicles, airplanes, industry, etc.) has dramatically increased the amount of CO^2 available to trap the Earth's infrared waves, thus turning up the dial on our warming blanket. This dial has fine-tuned and adjusted naturally over the millennia, usually (with the exception of a sudden natural or astronomical event) giving nature ample time to adapt to temperature changes at the surface. This is now occurring over just decades, fast forwarding the evolutionary process to where ecosystems may just fall apart if any key links are unable to cope. Again, mankind has altered the status quo.

Remember, it is not Earth's natural infrared waves that are stressing you in. The combined natural energies of the sun, Earth, and atmosphere produced and stored just enough infrared energy to provide a warming blanket that has given all of us the opportunity to survive on this planet…until mankind changed the status quo. From an environmental standpoint, please heed the warnings of the caring people who are passionate about maintaining the natural balance of our planet. Even if, coincidentally, we are headed into a natural cycle where Earth's infrared blanket becomes warmer, we don't need to accelerate the process by adding fuel to the fire. In this case it's fossil fuel. Read and educate yourself about this "greenhouse" effect. As you are now beginning to understand, everything you do does matter! So at least take gradual steps to address this issue within your means.

Since we all radiate infrared and our bodies sense infrared from other people, these waves are one example of energies that come into play when it involves the topic of "waves of humanity" that we will discuss in Chapter Five. There are parallels between our Earth's thermostat – our atmosphere, and your body's thermostat – the tiny neighborhood within your brain known as the hypothalamus.

As the atmosphere "regulates" its temperature by filtering and processing Earth and space energies, including infrared, so does your hypothalamus regulate your body temperature in addition to filtering and processing incoming energies from everywhere in your nervous system. As Earth's atmosphere generates energy in the form of lightning, clouds, and many more esoteric processes, so does your hypothalamus generate energy in the form of neurotransmitters and hormones to control many vital processes within your body. As our atmosphere becomes overburdened with excess energies (such as CO_2 from burning fossil fuels), it sends a warning "symptom", if you will, that Earth experiences as climate change. If your hypothalamus becomes overburdened with "stress energies," it also sends symptoms to inform you that your body is not at ease.

Many of you (actually tens of millions if not hundreds of millions) experience daily symptoms of such a core stress energy imbalance but have never been educated as to this vital link! You will shortly learn how this works and, most importantly, how to naturally rebalance this control center of your neighborhood.

CHAPTER FOUR

THE SLEEPERS MUST AWAKEN

Did you know that every *body,* including yours, strives to harbor a beautiful mind? A beautiful mind is benevolent and loving; always maintains a sense of good purpose; is always looking to inspire; does not respond with anger; is free from guilt and fear; can navigate the fine line between selfless and "self-first" without ever being selfish; and has absolutely no traces of greed, jealousy, oppression, intimidation, possessiveness, or ungenerosity. We are all moving along the same "staircase of time" from day one of our existence to achieve this goal. When a critical mass of people reaches this goal, there can be "Health on Earth"...even in your lifetime! Thus, our collective human energies do affect each and every one of us.

You may be asking, "Why a staircase of time?" Actually, it is a double spiral staircase, and this understanding is so important that I will expand on the metaphor.

People have, over the centuries, described the fabric of humanity in a variety of metaphorical phrases or passages. A most simple and beautiful one reflects that we are all branches on the same tree, reliant on the same natural energies for our sustenance. Thus, coexisting in harmony and cooperation, rather than in competition with each other, is the only strategy for keeping the tree healthy and fruitful.

Since you are now becoming more in tune with your energetic nature, let's be consistent and continue with our theme of your neighborhood. Most of you know that your DNA is your blueprint that orchestrates the structure and function of your physical body. Truly, DNA is your **D**ivine **N**atural **A**lly within. You may have learned from biology class that its structure is a double helix – two spiral staircases connected by energetic bonds.

Every one of your cells is a miniature ecosystem. The integrity of your cells is profoundly dependent on the natural vibration and resonance of the quarks and electrons that comprise your DNA. If anything changes the status quo and your DNA becomes stressed-in, cells will follow suit and your body will ultimately reflect this state of dis-ease. Earth is also an ecosystem, and, whether or not you are willing to accept the responsibility, the integrity of this ecosystem depends on human beings – all of us – living in harmony with the vibrations and resonance of nature! Picture each of us moving along a complex double staircase of planetary DNA, and Earth reflects the vibration of the whole structure.

Here's the problem. When you look at the reality of the current worldwide state of people's thoughts, words, and actions, there are obviously too many people sleepwalking along the staircase! In essence, there are too many dissonant minds generating enough stress energy to keep the balance tipped out of our favor. Earth is reflecting our energetic structure molded by our thoughts, words, and actions, and this has manifested as a decline in the quality and quantity of our vital resources (food, air, and water) in addition to fragmentation of families, communities, and countries. A particularly ominous warning sign is that some of our most important allies in nature, specifically the bees, bats, and even aquatic life (e.g., coral reefs), are struggling from the effects of our technology and the current vibration of humanity. All of these factors directly or indirectly stress you in.

At this moment in time, the double helical staircase still cannot act as a template for Health on Earth, as personal, societal, and cultural influences have fostered an environment where minds (from early on in life) become laced with fear, anger, guilt, prejudice, and greed. This, in turn, cripples one's ability to move toward a beautiful mind and optimal health. Yes, I am saying that many people have a mind that is lean in beauty and, in fact, often downright dissonant. It is reflected when someone's mind generates negative energetic thoughts, words, and actions, which I call lean-spirited energies. It reflects some degree of emotional and spiritual immaturity in every case.

We have all generated and been subjected to lean-spirited energy during our lifetimes. Lean in spirit does not mean absence of spirit! It means that one is momentarily or chronically struggling to gain traction and find their proper position on the staircase and is subconsciously crying out for assistance!

Many of you are sleepwalking along the staircase, unable to see that you are plowing into others, using an alternate blueprint as your guide. A sleepwalker cannot form solid bonds necessary for energetic integrity. However, the sleepwalker can awaken!

Lean-spirited energy from another person can stress us in only if we do not recycle it properly! In other words, a negative energetic influence can be recycled to a positive energetic influence – a "greening" of emotional energy, so to speak!

Since people are moving at different speeds towards a beautiful mind, and we cannot force change, how do we keep it from stressing us in while also helping others to wake up and elevate their level of maturity? Again, your perfect body to the rescue. Let's proceed…

CHAPTER FIVE

WAVES OF HUMANITY

The motion of emotion…

We now come to the energy-in-motion that reflects your degree of emotional maturity at any point in time during your physical life. That is, emotional energy that you choose to emit from your mind, and the waves of emotion that your body generates. Yes, your body generates its own emotions! For many of you, everything you thought you knew about emotions, feelings and symptoms is about to change.

Did you know that when you interact with people and experience their words and actions, your body senses, processes and collates all of the incoming energy of the experience a fraction of time before your mind becomes consciously aware of what is happening?

For example, let's say you are interviewing a person who has just crossed the finish line after running a marathon. You can see them, hear them, and feel their body heat only after your eyes, ears, and skin sensors have already processed the light waves, sound waves, and infrared waves and converted them to signals that were relayed to your brain. What about a more subtle situation, as when someone is approaching you from behind to give you a startle? What is that sense of generalized uneasiness before you even know someone is around? In this example, your body sensed and processed various components of that person's energy spectrum to give you cues to their presence.

The significant question remains, what was the contribution of the components of that person's human energy spectrum that generated these cues? Was it a subliminal shadow and/or sound? Was it a subtle change in the air temperature behind you, whether warmer or cooler? Could it be an effect of that person's brain waves? Were some free-spirited electrons at play again? Is it possible that our body has a greater sensitivity to each other's gravitational pull than we have been led to believe? The number of possibilities is mind-boggling, or I should say, "mind-vibrating."

Since your body processes the incoming energy before it comes to mind, then only your body knows the exact flavor of your experience! As we also obviously need to consciously know what any experience represents so that we can respond appropriately and in everybody's best interest, how do you think your body shares this knowledge with you? Let's go back to the example of when you sense someone is in your vicinity before you "see" them. What we often say in response is, "I had a feeling someone was near." There's the answer! You had a feeling. The flavor of any experience is shared via a vibration that we know as our feelings! **Our body emotions are our only true feelings and it all occurs in a fraction of time. I refer to this as the moment of truth.**

Your body always accurately communicates the truth, whether it senses the most joyous influences or the most lean-spirited energies. Thus, your body emotions are natural helpful vibrations that we must experience for our well-being. You must never suppress them or debate their existence. That would be a recipe for dis-ease, as you will learn. In fact, your body wants you to respectfully respond to your true feelings as they arise, especially when your body red flags a lean-spirited situation for you.

For example, how many of you have spent years or even decades stuffing your true feelings for fear that by responding with honesty, you could not prosper, you would "lose" something, or possibly that you would hurt someone's feelings? This is tragic and is totally out of sync with your body. If you are one of many people who are experiencing chronic symptoms of unclear cause, you may soon understand why. And, by the way, **feelings cannot be hurt…they can only be felt or recycled.**

How about those of you who are never shy to respond to situations? Does that mean that you have become a master at reading your own body language? Unfortunately not, because many of you allow your mind to distort your true feelings before you respond and, thus, your response is still out of sync with your body.

Question: What if your physical life depended on performing a task that required you to read and interpret the meaning of a short story, but when you began reading, you noticed that someone had inserted letters or symbols from a language that was totally foreign to you and even crossed out words and sentences and replaced them with gibberish? It would be frustrating. Why would anyone do that? What if that someone were you? It certainly doesn't make any sense that you would pick up the book, scribble all over it and then try to interpret it. Well, that's exactly what you are doing when your mind inserts certain specific negative energies when you are trying to read your own body language.

So, before we discuss the fine points of your body language and how to respond in the best interest of all, I must be sure that you know how to stop scribbling on your body's emotions!

Would you mind getting out of your way?

Energy-in-motion generated by your own mind of thought

First, you need to be clear on the following point: your brain is not your mind. The brain is part of the body. Your mind consists of patterns of vibrations within your brain that *you* choose to generate. Essentially, your human brain gives you the opportunity to develop a beautiful mind. Remember, we are mammals but we are not animals! The energy-in-motion from your mind is what you should refer to as your waves of thought. In contrast to body emotions that are always helpful, you now know that some thought wave energy can be classified as a negative energetic influence.

Most of you have seen a drawing or animation of an antenna with its radio waves rippling out in all directions. Think of your mind as a transmitting antenna, and your thoughts are the ripples of energy. This is a very accurate metaphor energetically. Since you are generating these energies, your body is the first to be affected by them and feels them the strongest! Thus, any negative blend of energy generated by your mind is most stressful to *your* body!

To put it another way, **you have no internal firewalls or energetic "non-stick coating" that will cause your thought waves to slide away from your own nervous system and into another person!** This may be one of the most valuable pearls of knowledge you will ever acquire.

There are three specific negative energetic influences that you must stop "transmitting" in order to be able to achieve optimal body health: anger, guilt, and fear. I call them mind-anger, mind-guilt, and mind-fear to drive home the point that they are inserted by *you* and not your body! These specific blends of unnatural waves that you choose to generate are inserted by you as an immediate reaction to a situation, as a response to a memory or thought of a past event or as you anticipate a future event.

In addition to their connection to the expression of lean-spirited energy, when you insert them or hold on to them, they are dissonant vibrations to your nervous system. In essence, these are broken records that will play over and over again until you turn them off. Thus, your body is forced to use its precious time and energy to recalibrate and rebalance…the very definition of stressing you in. So, what do these "mind waves" really represent?

Let's proceed…

The fine line between "com-passion" and anger

Anger is a judgmental expression of disapproval which carries overtones of "shame-on-you," vindictiveness, or resentment. At the extreme end of the anger spectrum we find rage. Unfortunately, anger has insidiously become regarded as a socially and culturally acceptable form of expression. Time to wake up! The link between anger, rage and body dis-ease is now very clear.

Thus, anger is not a natural wave of humanity, and any way you slice it, it has the potential to manifest grossly as dis-ease. When you insert anger as you immediately respond to any situation, it will, in addition to stressing you in, often induce a lean-spirited response by you towards another. A lose-lose proposition. Continuous waves of anger generated toward a memory of a past event also stresses you in big time – it really is bad for your body. Don't think for a minute that it is effecting revenge on the person who had done or said something that was lean-spirited.

On the other hand, as you will learn when we discuss how to respond to all situations in the most healthy way, if you can leave anger out of the equation, you will naturally generate *compassion* (used as a term to describe *com*munication with *passion*) as a response, which clearly allows for your freedom of expression, but is nonjudgmental and focuses your goal on waking up a person to the dissonance of what they said or did. It's a win-win-win for you and them because you did not insert anger (which stresses you in); you addressed your feelings through honest communication; and you may well have awakened the "sleeper," which will ultimately help you as well!

Did you know that by inserting and holding onto anger towards somebody, you may as well be angry at every individual or situation that has ever shaped that person's mind, including every ancestor back through the millennia? This applies across the spectrum, from the mildest situation to the extremely lean-spirited.

For example, suppose you discover that your bookkeeper has been surreptitiously tapping into your company's funds for their own personal use. You learn that this person is "self-medicating" their loneliness and stuffed emotions with gambling and alcohol use, and is using the company's funds to support these self-disrespecting activities. Yes, this employee's action violated your business bylaws, and whether one is "asleep" or not, one is ultimately accountable for one's actions.

However, who is really "responsible" for a mind that initiates a lean-spirited action? The parents who may have struggled with expressing love to this child? The person attempting to vent anger by bullying this child on the grade school playground? How about the doctor still practicing according to the old paradigm, who prescribed anti-anxiety medication to this person without taking the time to address the true emotional root of the anxiety symptoms? What "tendencies" (the epigenome) have been passed on through the ages that could add to the life challenges of this person? The list never ends.

Thus, when you insert and hold on to anger, you are, in reality, wasting your energy on an infinite chain of past events that you cannot change! What's done is done. Although the laws of a society provide guidelines for compensatory and/or punitive action for various lean-spirited actions, the people involved almost never explore avenues of healing bonds because, you guessed it, people tend to continue to hold on to anger. This is compounded by the fact that the "legal system" thrives on building firewalls between people, which further breaks bonds (which is a topic for another place and time). Anger really does cause you to misread your body's emotional message.

It is vitally important to remember that leaving anger out of the equation does not diminish your ability to respond passionately to a situation. In fact, you must respond in some way when your body sends a feeling that something is bothering you; otherwise you end up stuffing your feelings. As we have discussed, this is a recipe for dis-ease. Moreover, leaving anger out of your response gives you the clarity to see the bigger picture, so that you can make decisions looking forward to the best possible outcomes for all…that is, you respond to awaken the sleeper to their struggles, with the goal of restoring bonds as opposed to breaking them!

Guilt

No matter how you slice it – remorse, compunction, or self-reproach – guilt is the energetic manifestation of convicting yourself of a crime you feel you have committed or a mistake you feel you have made. The distinction between crime and mistake is very important, because the people who seem to be the most prone to insert chronic guilt are the ones who are more sensitive to others, more prone to second-guess themselves, and more likely to elevate an honest mistake to the status of a crime.

On the other hand, the person who plans and then commits a crime of harm, theft, or otherwise is more likely to insert no guilt whatsoever. What is wrong with this picture? The guilt card, or "chip," is certainly a paradox, in that the people who care most about not "hurting" others end up stressing-in their own bodies by keeping the guilt record playing. These chronic waves of constant second-guessing and self-doubt are very agitating to the body. It's as if you are beating yourself up. Not good. In addition, no one can make you insert guilt, nor put a guilt trip on you. So always remember, **no person can send you on a guilt "trip"; only you can insert a guilt "chip"**!

One shade of guilt energy can cause your mind to believe that a lean-spirited remark directed to you is actually the truth, which then forces you to stuff your body feelings and not respond to them at all! A most difficult aspect for the many sensitive people among us is related to you demanding of yourself a standard of achievement and caring that is unrealistically high so that any hint or suggestion of inadequacy causes you to devalue yourself and question your own competency. Holding onto guilt in this manner is especially prevalent among those of you who have been told earlier in your lives that whatever you do is not good enough.

For example, let's say that you are a woman who has a small child, who joins other moms with small children for a play group. Your child is playing with a toy and another child wants to play with it, but your child won't give it up just yet. The other mother comes up to you and says, "If you were a better mother you would have taught your child to share." This is totally lean-spirited and calls for immediate honest communication. But you expect so much from yourself that you dismiss your body's request to respond and decide that it is best to say nothing.

You're already reeling, when another mom asks you where your son goes to nursery school. You say that he doesn't go to nursery school. She says, "Don't you want him to get a head start on school, because, you know, kindergarten is very demanding these days." Again, this calls for honest communication as you know he is very advanced because you work with him at home. However, this just reinforces your misconception that you possibly made the wrong choice to keep him home, and you again allow guilt to override your inner sense that you should respond.

A few weeks later you discover you are pregnant again but you then have a miscarriage, which you wonder if you could have contributed to. Shortly thereafter you develop symptoms of fatigue that your doctors can't explain. Your husband tries to be supportive by saying he will do what he has to do to get you back to the "old" you, which unfortunately makes you think that you are now not an optimal wife. You are punishing yourself for a crime you did not commit.

From a divinely historical perspective, as many have said over time, just as you shouldn't falsely accuse your neighbor, you should not falsely accuse yourself, as you are bearing false witness against yourself! When the woman in the story above stops generating these waves of guilt towards herself, she will then read her body's message accurately, which will allow her to respond to others in a more healthful way, and any symptoms specifically related to her guilt and the stuffed emotions will begin to ease.

Thus, for all of you who have allowed this shade of guilt to block you from seeing the good heart that you have within, please remember the following: If you are someone who is constantly struggling with whether you are a "good" parent, child, or spouse, then you *are* most likely to be or become a "good" parent, child, or spouse, because you are conscious and aware of the importance of healthy bonding. It is just that you have been conditioned to believe that the happiness of your closest loved ones is totally dependent on you making perfect decisions. This is just not true. So lighten up on yourself. You will soon have new clarity regarding the subtleties of relationships!

Another shade of guilt involves any time you awaken to the fact that you have generated words or actions that truly call for an apology. Every one of us has had times where we have not been "full of thought" – not thoughtful, or not "full of care" – not careful. More accurately, as we have discussed, these are times where we have had a lapse in healthy consciousness (fallen asleep on the staircase, so to speak). Since you now know guilt energy stresses you in, this is now not an option.

To keep from inserting the guilt chip, there is a specific formula that is not complex. That is, as soon as you recognize that you have had a lapse in "healthy consciousness," it is important to apply the following:

> 1) As long as there was clear cause and effect, apologize as soon as possible! Do not make a decision to apologize based on the dramatics (or lack) of the response by the other person or people. Just use your newfound clarity to examine the facts exactly as they are.
>
> 2) Remember the lesson from the experience. (You will be more "awake" next time.)
>
> 3) Do what you can do, within your means, to commit your time and effort to "restore" any energy that was "displaced" by your action, that is, to make amends.

We all know that the person or people on the other end of your apology may well insert anger and generate ways to try to get you to insert guilt. (Are you beginning to see the negative ripple effects of these mind energies?) This may come in the form of "you should be ashamed of yourself," or "you should feel really guilty," or "you ruined everything," or "I do not accept your apology," etc. And remember, watch out for crocodile tears, so to speak, from the other person in an attempt to induce you to insert guilt. Usually, the drama is out of proportion to the situation.

The bottom line: No one can send you on a guilt trip unless you choose to go! Here is a template for a response that will help you:

> "I realize that I was not careful/thoughtful and I must be accountable for my action(s); however, I will not punish myself by feeling guilty or ashamed since it doesn't help anybody involved. Let's discuss how I can restore the energy that was displaced by my action."

Catastrophic guilt

I use the term "catastrophic guilt" to describe situations where one loses the chance to apologize conventionally. It involves a loss of physical life. We will shortly discuss the significance of looking forward to the best versus looking forward to the worst. However, when the mind decides not to look forward to the possible consequences of certain actions or inactions, it is an accident waiting to happen.

For example, if you operate a motor vehicle after ingesting alcohol or another brain-altering substance and another person loses a life, your action has literally led to the collapse of their neighborhood and has rendered all of their physical bodily energy and force useless to contribute their gifts to humanity. The displacement of energy is so great it is impossible not to insert guilt. This guilt can be released only if you passionately pursue an understanding of the higher (spiritual) influences, which will be discussed later in the text. Otherwise, your body will never be at ease. This is true for any similar case where, even if you had not planned or "intentionally" set out to harm another, your action or inaction resulted in the loss of the physical life of another.

Fear is a four letter word…

How many of you have assumed or have even been taught that fear is a natural emotion, courtesy of your body physiology that is here to protect you? This is false. Energetically, fear is an unnatural blend of mind energy that is in a class by itself when it comes to stressing you in. The reason you may be confused is that you know your body has a fight or flight mechanism, and you have equated this with fear. The truth is, they are energetically light years apart in what they represent to your neighborhood.

Fight or flight is a body emotion that prepares us to quickly defend our body (fight) or remove ourselves from a situation (flee) in response to a true threat of imminent physical danger. Our body doesn't create these vibrations so that we will be paralyzed with fear! It wants us to be fully alert to protect its physical integrity. Thus, your perfect neighborhood has no fear…only your mind does.

Fear distorts your body language in many ways:

1) Fear can cause you to internalize your feelings.

2) Fear can cause you to insert anger and rage.

3) Fear energy will lead to a sub-optimal result for any task that you perform.

4) Fear tampers with your unique energy spectrum and dims your true life glow energetically. In essence, you change yourself from a shining star into a dim bulb. People won't see the true you, and you will never be able to attract the people who really resonate with your natural glow.

Consider what happens when people (many of you) experience symptoms prior to speaking or performing in front of an audience, in addition to those who get symptoms before a written exam, interview, or manual task. The clammy cold hands, racing heart, and "butterflies" are your body's way of revealing to you that you have inserted fear energy! This is an awakening nudge from your neighborhood to release this fear. If this can happen from this common episodic situation, then imagine what chronic fear can do to your neighborhood.

Is it natural to have concern at times? Of course it is. Concern is our mind's use of available information that we normally use to keep our radar on potentially challenging situations.

Worry, on the other hand, is your mind's request for more information beyond the radar screen. We all worry from time to time; however, chronic worrying stresses you in, as this is a minor shade of fear. We all know someone who is a "chronic worrier." You will not find one who can honestly say that their body is at ease. Worriers know the truth of this.

Fear is your mind's construction of worst case scenarios and/or sub-optimal results, deflating your energy stores as you dwell on future "what-if's" and the potential for misery, morbidity, and/or mortality. First of all, since fear energy stresses you in, it immediately undermines the chances for the "best" result. So inserting fear is immediately counter-productive.

Second, as you develop a more beautiful mind, you will understand that "misery is optional," and you will be much less inclined to insert fear even in the most challenging of situations! If you presently cannot grasp that understanding, you can begin by asking yourself how some people with the most challenging life circumstances can stay afloat and claim to have no misery, while someone who seems to have everything "society" says is important can describe having feelings of deep misery? **Thus, it is** not the challenge that stresses you in, it is your waves of worry and fear that lead to body dis-ease and symptoms!

You may now ask, "Is positive thinking the answer?" No! The term "positive thinking" is a step in the right direction but falls short on many levels. "Looking forward to the best" is energetically superior to "positive thinking." In fact, it's best to avoid using the terms "positive thinking" or "wishful thinking." Those terms actually distract you from the reality of the situation. Looking forward to the best that can happen keeps you *looking* as the situation evolves so that you can react and adjust with a calmer clarity to changes ongoing in addition to gaining knowledge and meaning from the experience. Even in a dire situation where things appear bleak, if you keep looking you have a better chance of finding a silver lining of good energy or an open door of comfort. You should really place this into your vocabulary, as it is more true and your body is more at ease with the truth.

As a gentle example, suppose your young child is playing in a soccer game and their team is not quite as athletic as the other team. Another parent says, "I'm going to think positively that they will win but it is most likely just wishful thinking." If this parent had to say that they are going to think positively, that implies that they were initially inserting a shade of fear about the situation! Why assume or predict anything since it hasn't happened yet! In fact, who ever said that winning a game is the best thing that can happen? Just say, "I am looking forward to the best outcomes for all," then relax and take in the moment, which allows you to look at the game objectively, even if the best result is that your child learned what it was like to play against better players!

A word about meditation: Meditation *cannot* release the stuffed energy of body emotions or be a substitute for positive energetic influences, such as a natural loving relationship or purposeful work or activities. However, it is wonderful for temporarily shutting off the broken record of negative mind thoughts so that the brain can experience time with the more natural soothing brain wavelengths and connect with the higher and more esoteric universal influences. It is *very* valuable in this way, so it is wise to strategically set aside some time for your brain to resonate in this regard.

To review, since everything is energy-in-motion, so are your thought waves. They ripple to you first and strongest. Keep the negative energetic waves of mind-anger, mind-guilt, and mind-fear out of your neighborhood so that your body can devote its precious resources to maintain natural balance and healing. *Always* remove them from the equation prior to making any decision or taking any action. You will always have more clarity.

Your body language

Body-emotions (your feelings) and symptoms

How many of you realize that you have spent so much time trying to read other people's body language that you have lost track of your own?

As I emphasized earlier in the text, you have one body…one vessel. Your body is energetically your closest friend. Your body is always honest with you, is nonjudgmental, harbors no anger or fear, and never tries to induce guilt. In essence, your body is always in spirit. It wants to be naturally at a perfect state of ease, so when any influence enters the neighborhood, it must send guidance so that you can determine what the visitor represents and how to respond appropriately to it. This guidance is communicated by feelings and symptoms.

Your feelings are your body's way of communicating what it sees.

Your symptoms are your body's way of communicating that it is not at ease.

There are two areas of the nervous system that are especially sensitive to emotional energy and are major paths for communicating guiding symptoms. They happen to be among the most complex and "wired" areas of our nervous system. One, that you have already been introduced to, is the hypothalamus, which is a relatively small region of the brain that, despite its size, is the master control of many body systems and pathways. The hypothalamus has a very tough assignment. To give you an analogy, think of trying by yourself to fly dozens of kites of all shapes and sizes, with strings of different lengths, all at one time without one ever falling to the ground...twenty-four hours a day.

The hypothalamus could be considered the most wired structure in our body. It is directly responsible for maintaining body homeostasis (keeping your body in optimal balance), and, thus, if it becomes out of sync, your body will definitely take notice. By the way, it is the master control of our endocrine (hormonal) system. It is also your body's major bridge between emotions and the physical manifestations of emotion.

The second most sensitive area of your nervous system is actually your *gut*, or digestive tract. You may not be aware that this area of your neighborhood is bustling with nerve cells and neurotransmitters, including serotonin. It is also a major center for your immune system. Many familiar expressions link "feelings" with the gut, as when we describe a gut feeling. Not unexpectedly, the gut has a direct line that relays messages to the brain and vice versa, and the hypothalamus "sees" these messages.

Your body emotions (your true feelings) are of two types. They are all purposeful.

Healing: The natural vibration that you experience as joy! These emotions are generated in response to naturally harmonic energetic and higher influences coming in from a variety of sources. I will discuss these sources in detail later in the text, as they provide necessary sustenance as you move along your path. Suffice it to say, the more aligned you are within the natural fabric, the more deeply you will experience joy.

Revealing: These body emotions **reveal** that your neighborhood has experienced the energetic influences of lean-spirited words or actions. Remember, lean-spirited describes words or actions, not a person.

So, you ask, what does a revealing emotion "feel" like and what is it guiding me to do? It cannot be described in words. Essentially, it is your sense that *"something is wrong with this picture."* Suppose a person consistently makes remarks directly to you that are clearly lean-spirited (e.g., facetious, belittling, judgmental, etc.). What many of us have been conditioned to think is that the person is bad, so we use terms like "hopeless" or "mean-spirited" to describe them. What your body is actually revealing to you is that this person has, at least momentarily, fallen asleep on life's staircase and needs help to refocus toward the goal of attaining a beautiful mind! They may be struggling, troubled, or otherwise not acting in spirit, but people are not inherently bad, nor are they hopeless or mean-spirited. In fact, please erase the term "mean-spirited" from your vocabulary. By definition, spirit = good and purposeful. There is no meanness to spirit.

Thus, in response to this revealing emotion, what your body is guiding you to do is to recycle this vibe in the form of a response that will ease your neighborhood *and* help the other person (the source of the lean-spirited energy) to "wake up" at the same time! This is accomplished through a type of response that I call "compassionate release." We will shortly discuss the "rules of engagement." Remember, if your body did not have the capacity to accurately (a moment of truth) flag lean-spirited energies, you would be going through life vulnerable and never be at ease.

In regards to any lean-spirited remark directed at you by another person, many of you may now be thinking, "If these revealing emotions cannot be described, why is it that I often experience my heart pounding and my muscles getting tense?" Actually, what you are describing are *symptoms*. For you, unless you have actually been threatened physically, your body is signaling you that you have inserted anger, guilt, or fear into the equation, *or* you have previously internalized (stuffed, swallowed, not released, etc.) so many revealing emotions that it is getting rather crowded, energetically, in your emotional brain – i.e., your hypothalamus, et. al.!

Every symptom is a message from the body that it is not at ease, and symptoms that are linked to revealing emotions are especially important to recognize. Think of your symptoms as your body's way of nudging you to take action. Although symptoms may not be pleasant, remember that your body is always on your side! If you hold any resentment toward your body, your body can never be at ease! This is not speculation.

Thus, vibrations of revealing emotions require a response that is most appropriate for the individual situation. You *can't* ignore it or just think it away, as it will leave its energetic imprint within. To drive home this point, here is an analogous situation that you are all familiar with:

1) Suppose you are walking and suddenly your body sends a symptom of sharp pain in your heel. You are well aware of the response your body is requesting. You stop, take off your shoe and sock, and inspect the area. You find a sharp object that punctured your skin and remove the object. Your body quickly reduces the

degree of pain symptom and gradually eases the symptom altogether. If you don't take the object out, it will lead to infection or worse. *Positive thinking it away, meditating on it, or ignoring it will not work.*

Your body is naturally consistent and does not work any differently when it comes to your true emotions! So, you ask, are you saying that a revealing emotion generated in response to another person's lean-spirited energy-in-motion can become a pin in our proverbial "Achilles heel"? Yes, if we do not acknowledge it and respond, it can actually become a "pin" in, you guessed it, our hypothalamus. In fact, if you make it a point (no pun intended) to visualize it as a pin in your emotional brain, you may be more likely to address it sooner than later.

So what happens if we do not respond to our body's revealing emotions or we try to ignore them, and thus, end up suppressing or keeping them stuffed in? Well, I have "good" news, uncomfortable news, and challenging news for you. The good news is that our hypothalamus/emotional brain gives us some initial signals that it is not at ease in the form of symptoms, by using its nerve pathways, neurotransmitters, and other neuropeptides.

The uncomfortable news is that these symptoms frequently come early in life in the form of anxiety-type symptoms such as palpitations, muscle tension, sweatiness, headache, and bowel irritability, among others.

The challenging news is that if we continue to consistently internalize our true feelings, a second wave of body symptoms will come, even after several years, and this often presents as various combinations of persistent fatigue, generalized achiness, or gastrointestinal symptoms. The number of doctor visits specifically related to these symptoms is staggering.

The problem has been, most healthcare practitioners have not been given a foundation of knowledge regarding the role of chronically held fear, guilt, anger, and suppressed body emotions in relation to specific symptoms and syndromes, nor is the healthcare system structured to encourage doctors to spend the time to explore these issues with you. Thus, although you should always see your physician for a medical workup when experiencing any chronic symptoms, always keep in mind that "unexplained" fatigue, pain, and gastrointestinal symptoms/syndromes are very often your body's request for you to take inventory of any dissonant emotional energy you have inserted or internalized.

You have already learned the importance of turning off the waves of fear, anger, and guilt. You must now learn how to respond to your true feelings to create even more "breathing room" for your body's emotional processors.

The way to release chronically suppressed body emotions is to commit to honestly and mindfully responding to a situation or person as you experience your true feelings. Compassionate release does not mean that you can't respond passionately and to the point. To the contrary, it is all about learning how to use passion compassionately, as opposed to anger or defensiveness, to express yourself, so that you respond with the best intentions for your own neighborhood and send energy back to the other person in a "greener" form! You will absolutely get the most informative response in return that will help to define the situation and/or ongoing relationship.

When responding with compassionate release, always use the following keys as a guide:

1) Respond without rage (rage will always stress *you* in).

2) Respond based on the truth of the situation, not on assumptions (in fact, please remove the words "assume" and "probably" from your vocabulary).

3) Be careful how you respond to hearsay or gossip! This will be a challenge for many of you, because you are conditioned to think, "How dare they say something about me?" As I will explain, you actually need to confront the person who has delivered and rekindled the words that you didn't hear directly from the original speaker.

4) Respond fully and to the point, meaning that the other person must hear directly *from you* that their words or actions came through as lean-spirited and they must know exactly what prompted this emotion. Do not send responses through another person! It is a lose-lose-lose situation.

5) Stay in the present! Unless you have figured out how to travel back in time, a reference to the past will almost always dilute the energetic strength of your response. In fact, more often than you may realize, a person will not even recall the event that you describe!

Before I present some examples of how to respond optimally to your body's revealing emotions, there are some additional rules that you should apply consistently as you engage people on a daily basis.

1) The only true imminently destructive threat to you from another person is if they actually threaten physical bodily harm. Thus, if you are a person who would entertain thoughts of or actually threaten physical harm in reaction to a non-physically threatening situation, then you have grossly misread your body's message. This always reflects a mind laced with fear, anger, possessiveness, and/or greed, which presents as rage. This will severely stress your body in over time. You will inevitably suffer crises that will leave you dangling perilously on the edge of the staircase. Please

read carefully the knowledge presented in the chapter on spiritual influences.

2) When starting your response to an emotion, refrain from using the words "you hurt" or "you made," such as in the phrases, "you hurt my feelings," or "you made me mad." These words imply that you are blaming the other person for hurting you, when in reality ***they have not hurt anything*** (remember, emotions or feelings can be felt or recycled, but they can not be hurt), and the suggestion of blame will put others more on the defensive. In addition, these phrases often enable people who are struggling within, as they thrive on control and "feeding" on other people's anger and guilt. Always remember, you have the energy now in the form of an emotion, and you have the control and power to recycle and release it!

3) Refrain from starting your response with "Let me tell you…" Again, the words "let me" imply that you are asking one's permission to express yourself, and this is actually a subtle enabling of their behavior. You do not need permission to express yourself with care and honesty!

4) Do not express your passion with the word "mad." This implies rage, craziness, and being out of control. You are totally in control. The only time where the letters m-a-d should come into play is to remind you to Make A Decision instead of agonizing over how to respond to every situation. How many of you agonize over every decision and end up stressing yourself in?

5) Try not to use the phrase, "Don't ever say that," or "Don't say that again." You can't control what someone will say or even do in the future, and it has a threatening overtone. Just

stay consistent with carefully expressing how you honestly feel, and you will be amazed at the information you will acquire about everyone in your life.

Here are some examples to live by:

Suppose you have been experiencing symptoms that the medical community currently classifies as irritable bowel syndrome. Millions of people actually do experience gastrointestinal symptoms that are significantly linked to emotional vibrations within the nervous system, including the nerve centers in the gut.

Say you have a cousin who, for years, has attempted to aim subtle and not so subtle comments in your direction that were lean-spirited, but out of fear of ruffling the family feathers, so to speak, you choose not to tell her that the comments came through as lean-spirited. You suppressed your body emotions every time. In fact, now you feel a tightening in your abdomen just thinking that she may say something else that is lean-spirited. Upon reflection, you begin to recognize that your symptoms seem to manifest or intensify at times when you insert worry or fear. In fact, when you reflect upon this even further, you realize that you worry about almost everything!

The next day you are in the store with your cousin and she picks up several bottles of antacid, saying she uses a lot of it. You ask her why she uses so much and she replies, "Because I don't want to be sick like you." You immediately experience a revealing emotion and abdominal tightening, but this time you respond, "You are my cousin and I love you, but what you just said was lean-spirited. If you are struggling with something, I would be willing to sit and listen." This is honest and the type of response that more accurately would answer your body's request. In fact, you immediately experience an easing of your symptom, which confirms your new insight about the direct connection between your emotions and your symptoms.

There are several important aspects to your response. Your response placed the emotion with what the cousin said, not directly at the cousin. You prefaced the statement with "I love you," which is always true to our inner self because every *body* and soul is lovable…even though every *mind* is not! Also, you didn't have to directly rehash the past to experience a clear release of emotional energy.

You will always get another response to your expression, and this will give you very valuable information. For example, what if the cousin said, "Oh. I'm sorry, I know that I have been venting on you over the years and it's time things changed," and then gave you a hug? That certainly would give you an immediate glimpse of the positive ripple that occurs when we stop enabling other's lean-spiritedness towards us. Or she might have said nothing, as if to ignore you. This could represent her insertion of guilt, or maybe she is speechless, not expecting your response. What if she said, "I'll say what I want when I want"? That's very revealing, because you now learn she is struggling more than you had realized. You never told her that she couldn't say what she wanted, yet her mind distorted your comment as being a threat. She misread her own body language.

Please be aware that this example is not meant to suggest that one step of alignment and emotional energy release through a single expression of honest communication will address all of the energy imbalance within your nervous system. In fact, we already know that the person in this example inserts anticipatory worry or fear towards almost every upcoming situation or engagement, and she may well have shades of chronically held guilt or anger that have led to additional suppressed emotions with other relationships. However, this one seemingly small step can release more internalized emotional energy than you may realize, and can absolutely be a catalyst for a cascade of aligned communication and sustained easing of symptoms as we field the emotional energy from all relationship challenges.

How many of you have had a sense that your chronic symptoms are linked to fear, frustration and internalized feelings related to challenging life situations, especially with those "closest" to you? Unless you have reason to believe that a person will respond with physical violence, expressing how you feel as you experience a revealing emotion will always lead to a clearer view of family dramatics, even in the most tangled of family webs. There will be fewer games and less enabling of lean-spirited behavior, and you will find out who is presently tuned in to your frequency and who is not.

Let's suppose you are married with young children. As you work to balance the responsibilities and obligations of a career, marriage, and parenthood, your spouse has become a bit critical and impatient with you if one thing or another was not taken care of. Your spouse also displays many habits that are very dissonant to you, and obviously has many internal struggles, including being totally unable to accept any constructive advice whatsoever without being defensive. All of these factors dampened your romantic energy towards your spouse, and a vicious cycle ensued when your spouse's words became more and more lean-spirited. It got to a point where everything that didn't go "right" was blamed on you.

You told your spouse how you felt about things but you were always met with defensive and oppressive words and actions. When you developed symptoms of muscle twitching and fatigue, and the doctors said it was stress-related, your spouse responded by saying, "Don't tell anyone that you have a stress-related illness…it's weak." A very lean-spirited remark…however, you just let the revealing emotion linger in your neighborhood. You wrote letters trying to explain that it's nobody's fault and that you needed to talk. No response. Because of having young children and worrying about your health, you felt somewhat trapped and just stuffed a ton of body emotions internally, *fearful* of what might happen if you mentioned the word "separation."

More years go by. You develop generalized fatigue, which lasts for an extended period of time, and you are told you have a degree of chronic fatigue syndrome. You then learn how your body has been warning you of its agitation all along, which appears to be the reason you have been experiencing symptoms. You decide to turn off the mind-fear and to finally speak the truth to release the bottled up emotions. One more time, you express your desire to talk about the relationship. This time the response is, "Ok, I'll listen." Quite a shift, wouldn't you say?

Is it possible that, by you removing fear from the equation, the energy shifted to where your spouse now sensed that declining to listen could mark the end of the relationship as it currently existed?

The foregoing is actually a true account! What would *you* say to begin this type of conversation? The dialogue that you are about to read may not be typical or conventional, but it made a world of difference in the lives of this couple.

You initiate the conversation:

> "Picture a hot air balloon in flight. This represented my search for a person with whom I could cultivate a closely bonded loving partnership and share a lifetime of emotional and spiritual growth. When I met you, the balloon landed and settled at a beautiful place, where I exited the balloon to travel with you.
>
> "A closely bonded loving relationship requires a resolute commitment to open, honest, and non-judgmental communication. Since you had been unwilling to dialogue for so many years, despite my loving requests that we do so, I had been ready to tell you, for some time now, that I was prepared to reenter the balloon and move on. But my fear of what you would say if I told

you how I felt, and the fear of family 'fallout' from your subsequent actions, kept me from expressing my feelings.

"I need to hear the truth. Are you willing to *adjust your mindset* towards me, and *trust* that if we are both patient we may be able to strengthen the bonds that are currently strained? Are you willing to do this?"

Your spouse responded first with anger and defensiveness: "It's not me, it's you." Second, with fear and threats: "I am going to tell my family about this, and tomorrow I am going to quit my job."

You replied with this:

"I love you, but since your answer to my question is clearly no, I need to create space between us to reflect, and to regain my balance. Are you willing to continue to work together regarding other facets of our relationship and mutual family matters during this transitional time?"

Since you did not display any fear or anger in response, you gave your spouse the best chance to awaken to the fact that this was a truth that could no longer be ignored. In fact, in this case, your spouse then said something quite unexpected:

"Maybe it has been me. I think I have just been afraid to deal with my own fears and resentments from the past and I have carried them into our relationship. I want to try to make it work."

Your spouse did, then, display a less dissonant mindset for a period of time, and the energy of the relationship did begin to shift towards a more natural state. However, this was short-lived, as your spouse was impatient and expected you to "hurry" and "get up to speed" with all facets of the relationship, even before your spouse was committed to a more beautiful mindset. In fact, your spouse seemed to be sure that the "balloon" was grounded and that it wasn't going anywhere, despite the return of the dissonant mindset and lean-spirited remarks. New traces of fear that you inserted did delay a follow up conversation for a while, but you again refocused and you then had a second conversation.

You say the following:

> "At this point, I need to create space between us to reflect and regain my balance. I love you, I am not angry and I do not regret any time we have spent together. Are you willing to continue to work with me, regarding other facets of our relationship and mutual family matters, during this transitional time?"

The response: "I can't believe this. I need to go away for a day to think about things."

What happened next may surprise you, but it really did happen. The spouse returned the next evening, and said the following:

> "I thought about what you said about mindset. I have been carrying the mindset that you don't love me, which is never true at the deepest level, and I had expressed anger towards you to vent my own insecurities based on my fear of rejection. How would I expect our relationship to look when I put out those negative vibes towards you? The moment I reflected on this, I stopped worrying about anything and I felt a sense of ease. Even if we can't recapture our deeper and intimate bond, and we no longer live together, I understand that there is no

good whatsoever in being vindictive and clouding every other facet of our relationship. It would be like cutting off my own nose to spite *your* face."

The story of this relationship will continue to unfold, but all symptoms have eased and both partners have regained more natural traction along their paths!

This true life account demonstrates the huge upside potential that occurs when fear and anger are removed from the equation. When lean-spirited actions are no longer enabled and space is created, this provides an opportunity for both partners to regain momentum on their path to a higher level of emotional and spiritual maturity.

It is very important to understand that this example is not meant to suggest that proposing a separation or an easing of marital bonds should be the first thought that comes to mind when faced with dissonance in a relationship. To the contrary, to use this particular case, the one partner was chronically generating lean-spirited energy and would not even acknowledge letters or requests to sit and talk things out. There was an obvious **"relation-drift"** occurring between these two people that had begun many years before.

I use this term, "relation-drift," to describe the time when two closely bonded people find that they are taking markedly different paths, at different speeds, towards their own emotional and spiritual maturity.

If you have a partner or friend who is struggling so deeply that you are the recipient of a flood of lean-spirited energy and your partner is unwilling to dialogue peacefully, then there is no further viability to the specific relationship you once had, as you cannot thrive in an environment of continuous dissonance. You can exist, but you will spend most of your energy fielding and recycling lean-spirited energy…at best, you will be treading water. Thus, there must be honest and mindful communication.

I know many of you have experienced similar situations with a relationship and that many are going through this right now. A fact of life…drifts happen! The good news is that you now know what a relation-drift represents, and that vindictiveness is not an appropriate response. If you and your partner can sit down and have truly honest, nonjudgmental dialogue, there will be a dramatically improved chance of rekindling a marital spark or a friendship, or at least there will be a chance of experiencing a more peaceful transition.

Can you ever totally release a person? No you cannot, because, energetically, we are all connected within the fabric of the universe. You can downsize the percentage of your time and energy devoted to an adult relationship, but you can never energetically break up. As you now know, a person's inner light may be hidden by their thoughts and actions, but it is always requesting love, nonetheless. Thus, it is always helpful to send loving thoughts their way regardless of the distance!

As more people begin to understand the truth about emotional body energy, mind energy, and higher influences as presented within this text, there will be a dramatic increase in the percentage of healthy relationships across the board!

Suppose you move into a neighborhood where there is no through traffic and that seemed quiet and peaceful, but you soon realize that many of the neighbors have dogs, and one home has three dogs that sit all day behind a side gate and bark at anyone who passes by. Any dog's bark happens to be very dissonant to you and really cuts through the silence of the street. Your wife, who is home during the day, expresses her concern to the dog's owner a few times and, after nothing is done, even leaves a note or two for the owner to know the situation is still not resolved. The barking continues so you go to talk to the owner. You have a conversation at their front door where the owner eventually says,

"Your wife is a little nutty; maybe she should take a tranquilizer and close the windows if she doesn't want to hear the dogs bark."

How do you respond to this?

a) Punch him in the mouth? Absolutely not! That breaks one of the rules of engagement, since you were not threatened physically. A lose-lose situation.

b) Say,

"I am incredibly disappointed at your disrespectful attitude and your decision to make negative comments to me about my wife. When you wake up from your dream, maybe then we can have a constructive conversation. The barking situation is now out of my hands and in the hands of the county."

This would be a response that clearly makes its point, but it is totally a reflection of you inserting anger into the equation. In addition, the fact that he would say what he did shows a degree of instability which could escalate into a threatening situation. You don't know him very well and he could be intoxicated or under the influence of another mind-altering substance. Thus, this response is an example of the energy of the old paradigm. It may release the energy of the revealing emotion, but sends it out without "greening it," so you negate its net effect!

c) Immediately turn around and walk away without saying anything. Although there are situations where this would be appropriate (since sometimes silence does "speak" louder than words), in this case it would not, because you are choosing to build a "firewall" instead of looking to create a bond and awaken the sleeper.

d) The best response:

"Man, I don't know you very well, but you are my neighbor, and I always strive to find win-win solutions to all situations. I am not angry, but I am passionate about this issue because, whether you know it or not, the noise of a fearful, defensive, oppressive, or lonely barking dog is actually a health hazard because it irritates the nervous system. I will drop you a line tomorrow with my thoughts about what I would do constructively to remedy the situation if I were in your shoes. In the meantime, I am going to search the county website to see if they have any helpful tips on how to approach this situation. And, by the way, I do not plan to ever tell my wife about the comments that you made about her."

See the difference? You got your point across that the barking was not just disturbing to you but that it is also a health hazard to the other neighbors. (It actually is a fact.) You were able to include the words neighbor, win, passion, constructive, remedy, and helpful, which all carry good energy because they were generated with good intentions. He also is well aware that you will come across information on the county website on how to file a noise complaint, so he won't be caught off-guard if you do place the situation in the sheriff's hands, and he may be more likely to find a way to compromise.

You may be wondering, "Why not say anything about what he said about your spouse?" It's actually very powerful that you did not, because it was energy that was directed at someone who wasn't there to hear it, so its negative energy is quickly dissipated. If you later tell your wife what he said, then you have actually fallen into the trap of becoming the spokesperson and instigator of an energy that no longer exists in its original blend!

Remember: stay in the present. Unless there is a physically threatening comment about a person and the person must be made aware, it is not optimal to reinvent the past.

Another take-home point is to remember that when you deal with unfamiliar people or strangers, you must always take inventory of how to safely respond. In this case, the barking is actually dissonant energy that will continue to stress you in no matter how much you try to ignore it. It is draining for your body. The situation must be remedied by some means. Every situation has its own unique twist, however.

For example, what if you are driving and a driver behind you thinks that you are going too slowly for his or her liking, honks the horn and then speeds past you, screaming angrily all the way. There is no upside whatsoever to insert anger or rage (which stress you in) or to speed to catch up to him/her so that you can confront. In this scenario, your revealing emotion can still be addressed and greened by sending out thought energy desiring that somebody in this driver's life will awaken him or her to the fact of what rage represents before they experience a catastrophic event along the staircase (or on the highway!). This is good energy.

It is really important to remember to send similar waves of thought whenever you find yourself inserting frustration about lean-spirited events that are reported at a national or worldwide level. Unfortunately, as you know, this includes almost everything that we see or read in the news. Every joule of your energy counts and influences others, regardless of how inaccessible you believe the person or situation to be!

Also, never confront a person if he or she is intoxicated. Their responses are too unpredictable, and they won't remember what you said anyway. Many people, including children, insert fear and frustration if confronted by an alcoholic parent or spouse, and may even experience "fight-or-flight." Thus there will be hours, days, and years of stuffed emotions. This is why so many people who have alcoholic parents or spouses are experiencing symptoms related to a core emotional energy imbalance.

Here is an example to reinforce your understanding of the pitfalls of trying to reinvent "old" energy. What would you say if a friend of yours said that someone on your recreational league basketball team told them that you were a terrible player and a loser? In the old paradigm, you would insert anger (which stresses you in) and probably prepare to carry this anger energetically when you are in the presence of this person. Thus, you have inserted anger against a past event and are projecting it into a future that has yet to be "written"! Not good.

In the new paradigm, you think to yourself, if I remove anger from the equation and stay in the present, what is the real issue at hand and where can I insert positive energy? Then, a bulb (or rather, a true light) goes on in your head and you can see that since it was your friend that brought this to your attention, then it is your friend that you need to respond to with helpful insight. Thus, to your friend you reply, "That guy in the gym is obviously really struggling, since any person who uses the word 'loser' to describe somebody has serious issues to address. But I will explain, my friend, how you took his bait." You can then point out why it is beneficial for your friend not to dredge the memory banks and bring back to life the energy of a past lean-spirited remark.

Unless one needs to be made aware of a remark that conveyed an actual physical threat, then rekindling the negative energy of his or someone else's words is most stressful to the body of the person doing the rekindling. Since nobody wants to act as a carrier pigeon of negative energy, your friend will think twice before he drops that "stuff" in your lap again!

Here is a very important word about words. Since everything is energy-in-motion, that also includes words. You have already learned the profoundly important fact that any energy you generate will affect you the most. The words loser, trash, idiot, stupid, creep, and jerk, to name a few, are negative energetic influences. We discussed how your neighborhood nervous system does not have a firewall or non-stick coating to deflect energy-in-motion. Thus, when you call somebody a loser, you are energetically calling your own body a loser, and this stresses you in!

Also, when you use these words, they are almost always preceded by a wave of anger that your mind inserted. Thus, your body is most strongly exposed to the thought waves that formed the negative words and the waves of the spoken words themselves that are carrying the anger. A lose-lose for you! Another person's body and soul are not the source of your frustration. It is a struggling mind or lean-spirited actions initiated by a struggling mind. A mind cannot be a loser, trash, or otherwise. A sleepwalker on the staircase may be a challenge, but you don't throw them off! They need help to regain their healthy consciousness.

A persistently struggling mind is a reflection of emotional or spiritual immaturity, very often due to an underexposure to good energy, love, and respectful knowledge anytime from the earliest moments of life through the present. So parents, please, please, please shower your children with good energy, love, and respectful knowledge. You can only do this if you, yourself, can recognize your own key imbalances and reconnect to all sources of good energy.

Speaking of children, how do you handle situations that present to you indirectly from your child? This is a very sensitive issue because children are often hesitant to confront. Suppose your son is in Little League baseball and it comes time for all-star selections. You believe your son is one of the top two players and there are two spots. Your son comes back from practice telling you he was not chosen and you insert anger into the equation. One of the two chosen is the coach's son and, of course, you cry "Nepotism!" Then you remember to turn off the anger and ask yourself what the true issue really is: what you feel about the coach's decision or how you feel about how your son feels! Of course, you are passionate, because your son may feel sad and disappointed! This is an opportunity to teach your son. So, you need to explore this with your son first.

You sit privately with him and say first, "So how did you feel when you first heard that you weren't chosen?" He might say,

> "You know, Dad, at first I felt angry and disappointed, but then I realized that those kids were about as good as I am and I really can't complain. I love baseball and it's not about beating someone out of a spot or being better than someone; it's about me working and practicing to be the best that I can be. Things will then work out the way they should in the long run."

After you pull your jaw up off the floor, you give him a hug and say, "You read Dr. Bornstein's book, didn't you?" He winks and goes outside to hit some baseballs.

Of course he may say, "I was angry and disappointed when he first told me, and I still am." The next thing you might say is,

> "Son, the decision has been made, but what if the coach came to you and said, 'It was a really hard decision to make and I wonder if I made a mistake. Could you help me out by making a checklist comparing you and the other two players in all categories from your perspective on hitting, fielding, pitching, base running, batting in clutch situations, and sportsmanship so I can compare it to my list to help me more closely evaluate my decision?' Would you do that, son?"

You could tell your son that if the list is positive to his side by +2 checks or more, you and he will go to the coach, without anger, to present how you feel, and maybe the coach won't make the same mistake next time.

You can fine-tune this approach based on your specific words, but the most important point is, your body was revealing that your passion should be directed to more about how your son feels than about a sports coach's decision. If your child has specific emotions, work with him or her to evaluate the situation behind the emotions, and if the situation was really unfair, figure out how he/she can address the situation in a comfortable way. Both your health and that of your child will benefit by not inserting anger and then working through a major life lesson!

The following example illustrates the importance of not assuming. Suppose you are carpooling to work and the other driver has been a bit late a few times recently, and you have barely made it to class/office. You talk to him and things seem to be straightened out. Today he is now 20 minutes late, and consistent with the old paradigm, you choose to insert anger into the equation. You really have to go, so you drag your spouse out of bed to drive you to work. You plan to talk to him when he gets to work. About a half hour into your normal commute route, traffic suddenly slows to a halt. Nothing is moving. You turn on the radio to find that an accident occurred 10 minutes ago and you will be blocked in for some time.

Now you are getting symptoms of muscle tension and a headache. You are thinking, if he just would have picked me up on time, we would have avoided this whole mess. You arrive at your office and notice that there are fewer co-workers than you would expect. Just then, your phone rings and you see the number is his. More symptoms (anger). You answer, and he says, "I am at your house and no one is answering. Are you okay?" "No. I'm not okay…I'm angry that you didn't pick me up on time, and

I got stuck in a traffic jam." He responds, "What are you talking about? It's Wednesday, and we always start work an hour later on Wednesdays. I actually came a few minutes early because I heard on the radio that there was an accident and I was going to take an alternate route."

Oops.... Always get the facts so you can confront appropriately! The driver could be struggling to follow through with his commitments and you may ultimately decide not to ride with him any longer, but he also could be on the way to the hospital with a heart attack. It will ultimately save you time, energy, and symptoms.

Thus far, I have presented just a few of the many possible examples of how important it is to keep anger, guilt and fear out of the equation when you experience your true feelings. Then you can respond with com-passion as you green and release the energy. This keeps your emotional brain, and the rest of your body, naturally at ease. In addition, you now know that it helps others to wake up and reflect on their actions to refocus and realign themselves along the staircase. Remember, we are all connected energetically, so what naturally helps others, helps you as well. Thus, we have the new paradigm of learning to green your emotions for the benefit of all!

I want to bring to your awareness a type of situation that is dangerous times two. It is a silent epidemic among humanity and many people are afflicted. There is a large subset of people who have "decided" very early in life that it is more comfortable to please all of the people all of the time as opposed to expressing how they feel as emotions arise. In fact, the mind reasons, if they could suppress the revealing emotions so deeply as to keep them from even barely entering their consciousness, they wouldn't have to deal with them at all. Since you now clearly know that the body's emotions arise prior to thought and must be dealt with, you can see the added danger in this scenario. Here are three examples:

1) After being treated for a very minor skin laceration, a man experiences an extended period of fatigue and weakness. His medical workup excludes any "measurable" dis-ease, so he is diagnosed as having chronic fatigue syndrome and has suffered with these symptoms for three years. He reads about how the emotional brain – the hypothalamus – could be involved. He makes a phone call. On being questioned, he says that everything else is 'fine' in his life – he is happy at his job, he is very easygoing, no conflicts, and he has never had an argument with his wife of seventeen years. This is a major red flag!

He may not have ever had an argument with his wife, but his body has certainly been piling up certain revealing emotions from her incoming energy from time to time. On further questioning, he says his "childhood was, well, my father demanded respect, but it was a normal household." This is another clue, telling us he may have some suppressed emotions regarding his relationship with his father.

At this time, his body was already on the verge of symptomatic dis-ease. The touch of dissonance from the minor injury just exposed it a bit earlier. It is guaranteed that his body will be more at ease if he learns to get back in touch with his emotions and starts responding to them.

2) A lady in her eighties comes in for general medical care. She had suffered a serious type of complication of polio earlier in her life, which caused her to lose most of the use of her legs at that time. She is very intelligent and she enjoys talking, thus much of her life history was revealed. She relates that since very early in life, prior to the polio, she "learned to control" her emotions due to some challenging and sad life experiences, so she rarely ever allows herself to release any emotional energy. In fact, she can't remember the last *year* that she cried!

This case raises a question relating to doubly stuffed emotions and dis-ease. Since immune system imbalances are inevitable when the emotional brain is chronically agitated, is it possible that this lady manifested the most devastating manifestation of polio in the nervous system due to years of suppressed emotions? Yes, it is not just possible...it is likely. It would be wise for the medical community to focus more attention on the role of emotional stress energy imbalance in relation to the manifestation and resolution of infectious dis-ease.

3) A young man is diagnosed with a condition called gastroparesis where the motility of the stomach becomes imbalanced. This condition is associated with various "classified" dis-ease states, but it also presents without any "obvious" cause. This man had no obvious known predisposing factors. On questioning, he revealed that he has always had to be the peacemaker, the "strong person," the calming force in his large family, and he stuffed a heavy weight of revealing emotions all of his life. This very, very insightful man then asked, "Could my nausea and vomiting metaphorically represent my body's way of telling me that I need to release this energy?" As he began to respond to situations more truthfully and naturally, his symptoms began to ease!

Again, physicians and healers should take notice that the main focus of twenty-first century medicine will be stress energy and its relation to symptom and dis-ease management. Your practice will become obsolete and stagnate in the realm of chronic dis-ease if you do not embrace this new paradigm.

We need to look very seriously at extremely lean-spirited human energy that takes advantage of the vulnerable among us. It always stresses in those at risk, and it always produces dissonant vibrations that cannot be released easily. This energy is the energy-in-motion from people who threaten physical harm repeatedly over an extended period of time. People who use this type of oppression or intimidation are also stressing themselves in on many levels, as you will see as you read further.

This type of lean-spirited energy-in-motion is generated by posing a continuous, ongoing threat of physical harm to a child or dependent adult, by verbally degrading or aggressively intimidating them. Children and dependent adults are ultra-sensitive and vulnerable, and have very little leverage to respond honestly. When a parent, guardian, or other person is degrading or intimidating, the body senses a true threat, and a revealing emotion of fight and flight is produced. Since the dependent or vulnerable often cannot fight or flee, this vibration becomes sustained. This is super agitating to the hypothalamus.

A child or dependent adult living under a constant threat of this type will suppress a huge amount of emotions, will almost always experience anxiety symptoms, and will have a significantly increased risk of developing secondary symptoms of a core emotional energy imbalance at an early age.

People who generate this blend of energy must awaken, as the negative ripple effect from this type of lean-spirited energy weighs heavily on humanity and is a significant barrier to achieving a critical mass of positive energetic influences necessary to achieve Health on Earth in our lifetime. For those of you who are the oppressor or intimidator (you know who you are), since you had never been given a benevolent foundation of knowledge to live by, your life experiences have led to a lean-spirited mindset that you carry forward to others. However, you are still accountable for your actions, and in more ways than you may realize. So, please, release your own deep wedge of fear and anger to respect and reconnect to your body and soul so that your mind can shift from being a source of inflammation to becoming a source of inspiration!

If you are one who actually moves to directly physically harm or destroy another person's body in the absence of a truly imminent, provoked physical threat, then you have totally fallen asleep along the path and, unless you take giant steps to heal your wounded mind and devote time to replace the energy you have drained from humanity as a result of your actions, your body will never be at ease. This is a reflection of extreme emotional and spiritual immaturity.

It is mind-boggling to think of how many people still act as if they own another person's body. Be aware that there are no "crimes of passion." There are crimes and there is passion. They are energetically far apart from each other. **There is no guidance in the universe that will guide you to physically harm somebody because a relation-drift occurred!** If a partner or companion chooses to ease away or develop other bonded friendships, then please be thankful for the time you were together and move on. This shows maturity. Other good energy and influences will come in to fill the "void" as long as you have this mindset.

CHAPTER SIX

IT'S GETTING ON YOUR NERVES

Dissonant energy-in-motion

The body always wants its brain to have optimally healthy focus at all times. Healthy focus means simply that your brain will be best able to guide you through the task at hand. Your body really is a most faithful advocate for you!

You may ask, "How is my brain focused when I am sleeping?" Well, did you ever reflect on the fact that when you are asleep, your brain is not? In other words, your brain is very focused on generating waves at a lower frequency to refresh your neighborhood. Thus, any distraction that occurs while your mind's antenna is "up" (i.e., when you are awake) will cause you to be less full of good thought (less thoughtful) and/or less full of care (less careful), and any distraction that disturbs your brain's focus when you are asleep will cause your sleep to be less restful!

The types of distractions that I am referring to are called dissonances. Dissonant means not in harmony. For you, it means that there are certain sounds, odors, visual stimuli, or other energetic influences in your environment that are always an energetic drain on your neighborhood and will always continue to be unpleasant to your neighborhood even if you think you have developed tolerance to them. They are distracting and literally "get on your nerves." There are more dissonances entering your space than you might possibly imagine…and on initial exposure, your body gives you a signal (symptoms) that it is out of its comfort zone so that you can act accordingly. The problem occurs when you adopt an "It's okay, I'll get used to it" mindset.

Let's discuss how your body helps you deal with dissonant energies. Up to this point, it should be very clear to you that your body is very consistent in its ways. You now know that, as opposed to the mind, the body doesn't take time to debate whether or how it should respond. It feels, reveals, and sends symptoms when it needs your assistance to heal! To preserve the brain's healthy focus, after your body immediately alerts you to the distraction (the wake-up call), if it senses that you are not doing anything about it, it then begins to recalibrate the core neighborhood to buffer the distraction so that your brain can continue on with optimal focus. But there is a price to pay…in body joules. Because you perceive the dissonance as less prominent, it may appear that you have adjusted just fine. Well, everything is not fine. Recalibration takes energy, which weakens your neighborhood, *and* there is often extra toxic baggage that comes with the dissonance.

Here's an analogy to start you off. Suppose you are at the beach and decide to go into the water. You wade into the shallows and notice that the water is very briskly cold. A wave quickly rolls in and momentarily covers your body. You all know the feeling when that happens…a gasp and the momentary muscle tension (symptoms). This is your body giving you a firm nudge (the "wake-up call") that it is not optimal to linger in this locale. Since you want to swim, you continue to stay in the water because, based on your past experience, you "know" that you will temporarily "get used to it" for a period of time as you swim in the water. As you temporarily feel more comfortable in the water, this is your body beginning to buffer the dissonance because (even though it was your choice to stay), the body must, *for your safety*, always work with the premise that you are unable to remove yourself from that locale! Even though you may feel more comfortable for a while, your neighborhood is pulling resources and working overtime to direct traffic within your circulatory system to protect your vital core and maintain focus!

Of course, you wouldn't choose to linger in the cold water for hours at a time…you know that would seriously threaten your body's integrity. The problem is, since most of life's dissonances are common mankind-generated energies and do not imminently threaten the neighborhood in a matter of hours, we have remained generally unaware of their stress-in effect.

We also need to be mindful that very young children may not be able to communicate their discomfort about dissonances in a specific enough way, which often makes it challenging for us to easily pinpoint the exact source of the dissonance. Thus, always keep in mind the fact that dissonant energies may be as dissonant, or even more draining, to a child's body than it is to yours.

Noise

"Noise" = dissonant sound waves. I am not talking about loud sound…we all know that enough decibels of any sound can stress your auditory neighborhood to the point of pain and even bond breaking. I am saying that noise does not have to be loud to stress you in. If you have any doubt that your body sends a wake-up call to dissonances, I have just one thing to say: fingernails dragged across the chalkboard. Spine-tingling symptoms, wouldn't you say? Now, of course, that is not an energy that you would ever have to deal with on an ongoing basis; however, if that were the case, yes, your body would make changes to buffer this over time.

Almost all noise pollution is directly or indirectly related to mankind. For example, most of you have been bombarded with the noise of motors, engines, machines, and electrical "hums" for so long that these distractions barely reach your consciousness unless they are painfully loud. Loud or not, your body still has to use joules to deal with every exposure. The noise of motorcycles, lawnmowers, airplane engines, and vacuum cleaners are common exposures that are among the most dissonant.

A residence near a subway track or airport is another example where tolerance is fooling you. You move in and every 30 minutes you hear the noise and feel the rattling of a subway car or plane. After several weeks you tell people you're so used to it that you really don't even notice it anymore. Sorry, your body continues to notice. Isn't it interesting that some communities near airports receive complete monetary funding to "soundproof" their homes! You may say that the sound of an engine or motor is music to your ears, but it is noise to your body. The purr of a cat represents ease. The "purr" of an engine represents dis-ease.

How many of you can't fall asleep without an electric fan turned on? Well, in addition to the unwelcome electromagnetic field that it generates, it is dissonant (*not* comforting) to your body. The fact is, you are using the fan to replace another dissonance that you don't know how to deal with! In the event that there is an even more irritating noise in the vicinity (i.e., city traffic, airport traffic, struggling noisy neighbor that has forgotten that we are all branches of the same tree, etc.), you may have to decide between the two dissonances, i.e., the fan versus the neighborhood noise, until you can address the situation.

However, many of you use the fan to drown out the dissonance of your own mind! In other words, at bedtime you insert worry and fear regarding the days events and are now worrying about tomorrow's challenges. You may even be inserting anger or guilt about the previous day's events. Using the fan for this reason is only serving as a band-aid, as these pins and even suppressed emotions are still embedded when you wake up.

Next is a very sensitive issue for many people – the bark of a dog. It is known that it is one of the most dissonant noises and one issue that clearly challenges our "Love thy neighbor" commitment. Are you aware that many dogs have descended from wolves that were bred to retain their juvenile characteristics and to bark a lot? This may have served people well through the centuries on farms where dogs actually had a residential purpose other than being "your best pal," and no one denies that dogs can be trained to be valuable assistants among certain groups.

However, all factors considered, a dog's bark is a net negative energetic influence when it comes to our modern closely-built residential neighborhoods. You may already have personally discovered that a neighbor's dog's bark is one of the few common dissonances that your body doesn't seem to want to buffer. Why do you think the barking is always consistently irritating?

The reason fits beautifully into your new understanding of your body. Follow closely. While your body does want you to maintain healthy focus, you have also learned that it always strives to harbor a beautiful mind! As you know, one component of a beautiful mind is compassion. A dissonant noise persistently generated by another living being almost always means that it is struggling in some way. A chronically barky dog almost always indicates a struggling dog, which, in turn, almost always indicates a struggling dog owner. Your true self always desires to help, and, thus, until the situation is addressed in some way, the dissonance will remain quite apparent!

What about a spouse or bedroom partner who snores? (No, it is not natural to chronically snore and this is actually a risk factor for more threatening dis-ease.) It is irritating to your brain while you are awake, and your body will absolutely continue to be irritated by it even when you are asleep. Your body wants your brain to focus on healthy sleep, so, you guessed it, your body buffers it, but only to some extent because snoring indicates a body that is not at ease. If you think you are sleeping through this noise, you are mistaken. It is known that the bed partner of one who snores may wake up dozens of times per night, whether they are aware of it or not. It is a risk factor for dis-ease in both the snorer and the "snoree," if you will. Thus, earplugs are never a long-term answer. Remember, it is the snoring that needs to be addressed, not the bed partner who is tired and needs some rest! You certainly would take action if your bed partner were awake and moaning or crying every ten seconds.

One of the most profound examples of our overriding sense of compassion involves the dissonance of a baby crying and the mother's sensitivity to it. What do you think are the two things that a baby's brain must focus on to thrive? No, not wetting the diaper or spitting up. Here's a hint: what are the two things a baby does best? The answer is sleeping and crying! Since a baby is totally dependent, crying is the only way to alert Mom that it is struggling in some way. Thus, crying must be a dissonance that Mom will not easily develop tolerance to. Since attending to the baby is a loving influence, the net effect despite the dissonance is profoundly positive. After nine months in the womb where Mom and baby bond with each other's frequencies, it is no wonder that mothers can often detect the distant cry of their baby through all kinds of distractions.

There is one other point that parents and expectant parents should keep in mind. Most of you have heard of ultrasound, an imaging procedure used primarily in the healthcare realm. Ultrasound produces ultra high frequency "noise" that we cannot hear but that our bodies can feel. When used during pregnancy to image the young life within the womb, this noise may be more dissonant to the young life than we realize and, in fact, it is possible that this noise *is* "heard" within the womb. As always, ascertain from your practitioner the exact purpose for any medical procedure and use a solid foundation of knowledge to weigh the potential risk vs. the benefit.

Joules to remember:

Do not get used to loud sounds...your auditory neighborhood can only buffer for so long before bonds break. Remember that noise does not have to be loud to stress you in. Do not ignore your body's wake-up calls. Instead, reflect with clarity on the reason for the "call" and respond with healthy focus. Realize that the "sound of silence" is not only golden, it preserves joules and will exponentially improve the energy and value of your community!

Dissonant odors

Odors are another energetic influence that we may think we have gotten used to. By the time we smell something, its energy has already moved through our olfactory neighborhood. One area of the body to where the scent receptors send messages is, you guessed it, the hypothalamus. As you know, your body can find an odor so dissonant that it sends the symptoms of headache and even nausea. Quite a wake-up call, wouldn't you say? Odors often carry toxic baggage. For example, say you are looking for a new residence to relocate to and you find an area that you like. As you stroll around the block, you catch a whiff of a dissonant odor, especially when the wind picks up. It reminds you of a refinery type of odor you sometimes smell as you drive along a highway or turnpike. You talk to the neighbors and mention this and they say there is a factory miles from here, but "after a while you don't even notice it anymore." Red flag! Where there is refining or burning, there is toxic energy and particulate matter that you breathe in with every breath.

What about second-hand smoke? It is always dissonant on first exposure…you may just not remember. With the known toxic baggage that goes along with cigarette smoke, are you surprised that cigarettes are scented in an attempt to mask the dissonance? Please do not be fooled by odors that are designed to mimic nature's scents. The body's message on initial exposure may be very subtle, but the wake-up call is still there! Many candles and most air fresheners are clear examples. These add toxic baggage. How many of you do not know what a real freshly cut lemon smells like? Lemon-scented products are not even competent fakes. Do you like that new car smell? Well, it doesn't like you.

Many people around the world burn incense. Just because incense is usually associated with meditative or relaxing venues does not mean that its smoke is relaxing to the body itself. It is in your best interest to know the source of its production and the ingredients, and to remain aware that all smoke contains at least some degree of toxic baggage.

Joules to remember:

To use a play on words that may help you to remember, our air is filled with "false *scents* of security." It is a fact that the more you avoid them, the more conspicuous they will become to you, and you will more promptly seek refuge from this "stress air"!

A taste of dissonance?

Although we often find ourselves with a scrunched-up face and an urge to expel the food from our mouth, the wake-up call to a dissonant energy that engages our tastebuds is often subtle when chemical fakes try to "slide" by. Artificial sweeteners, such as aspartame and sucralose, try to con your buds with sweetness. Sucralose is a sugar molecule that is forced to bond with chlorine molecules! Aspartame, found in many diet sodas, doesn't even resemble a carbohydrate at all…in fact, it more resembles a protein, as two amino acids are forced to bond. Thus, they stress you in and have the potential to contribute to more serious disease. There are many, many people who, on first exposure (e.g., to a carbonated beverage), can instantly recognize the dissonance of these so called artificial sweeteners. It is clear to many that there is something wrong with this picture. For the rest of you, why are you ingesting this? If you want to release body mass, apply all of the restorative knowledge within the text and you will ease to your healthiest mass!

Also, our tastebuds are insidiously exposed to other dissonances so early in life that we often become unable to enjoy nature's best food without them. The gustatory dissonance that processed food brings into our life from an early age is primarily the overabundance of added salt. Yes, our bodies require sodium and chloride to survive, but we should strive to allow our bodies to extract and absorb the sodium it requires from nature's finest foods, naturally…not force-feed it a version that is concentrated out of proportion to nature's best. Most of you have been buffered to the higher salt diet so you find low-salt foods very bland. Because of this, you may not have ever experienced the true natural flavor of any of nature's finest.

There is an abundance of resources that list the highest added sodium foods. Isn't it interesting that food suppliers are offering an ever-increasing number of products labeled "no added salt." Begin to chip away at this issue at a comfortable palatable pace for you. Your body will love you for it.

Joules to remember:

Be knowledgeable about what is sliding by your "buds." Chemicals and concentrated extracts that are supposed to be flavor enhancers are actually flavor reducers, holding you hostage, and we haven't even discussed the baggage that your body has to deal with once these energies gain access to your neighborhood. Respect your body and it will respond in kind!

The dissonance of living space

Clutter in your immediate surroundings literally gets on your nerves. Yes, your body buffers this too, at your expense. When dealing with clutter, this is one time where you should be "m.a.d."! Not mad in the energetic sense of anger or rage, but Making A Decision mad. How many times have you had to squeeze by that box in the garage or stepped over that same pair of shoes on the closet floor. How many of you are literally tired of seeing all of those collectables covering every square inch of counter space or even experience an uneasy feeling every time you pass your cluttered desk?

Here's what you need to do: Tomorrow, choose the space that seems to bother you the most. Take a moment to scan the space as if this were the first time you ever saw it. In this new light, you will see everything that is wrong with this picture. You will wonder how you let this go on for so long. Smile inside and say, "I should be m.a.d. (making a decision) about this now." Then begin to de-clutter the space. Once the space is appropriately re-organized with the items that are most purposeful for you, if you have "leftovers" and have absolutely no other appropriate space for them, then you must learn to release! I know that many of you attach sentimentality to everything you have, if only the tiniest sliver of it.

Release is good if it has a good purpose. Find another person on the staircase of humanity…the items that are not presently essential to you may indeed be of great use to someone else!

You may ask, "How do I get my children to de-clutter their rooms?" Well, it is important to teach them early that clutter actually drains their energy, and the energy it takes to de-clutter will actually give them more energy in the long run. Kids love to hear the words "more energy." However, please make them aware that being tidy does not mean everything has to be in perfect order and spotless.

Since clutter is ultimately the result of accumulating too much stuff, you should expand your use of the "should be m.a.d." paradigm to every time you are planning to make a purchase that is going to compress your living space. In other words, if you are shopping, browsing, or otherwise, as soon as you take out your currency or begin to enter your credit card number online, stop, and think to yourself, "I should be mad"…then give yourself a minute or two to review what you have in your hand or shopping cart. First ask yourself truthfully, "What is my purpose for buying this?" You will be surprised at times what the answer is. Then if you do confirm its good purpose, when you bring it home, or receive it in the mail, think of something equivalent that you already have that can be donated or recycled, to create space for your new acquisition! This is good.

Joules to remember:

If you visualize all of the dissonances you are chronically exposed to as tiny pins on your brain's bulletin board causing vibrations that agitate your nervous system, you will be more likely to address them early to help your neighborhood. And remember, every intermittent or persistent dissonance costs your body, depleting your store of energy, joule by joule. Does this mean that you have to immediately have your snoring spouse sleep in another room or that you have to quickly move from a noisy neighborhood? Not necessarily, but start getting things off the list! Do not assume that one particular situation is necessarily the deepest pin. A situation that you think is minor may actually be a large pin of agitation and vice versa. For example, a cluttered desk may stress you in much more than a large cluttered garage, and you may not know this until you de-clutter and do your paperwork.

Thus, no dissonant energy is necessarily minor in influence. Just get things off of the list whether it would be by care-fully confronting, de-cluttering a space, or making a decision with all available information and then looking forward to the best! Your body will love you for it.

Please remember not to tell people that *they* are dissonant or getting on your nerves! Rather, when appropriate, just care-fully bring to their attention what the dissonance is. For example, suppose you are sitting at the dinner table and you feel a constant vibration of the table. You become aware that it is coming from a person with a "restless" leg. It's not best to say, "Excuse me, could you stop your leg from shaking? You are getting on my nerves." It is more appropriate to say, "Excuse me, are you aware your leg is shaking a mile a minute?" If they reply, "Yes, and you just have to deal with it," that reply is lean-spirited, and you can carefully respond as appropriate for the situation. More often than not, they will say, "Sorry (or, "Thanks for telling me"). I don't even realize it's doing that." There are many similar examples.

The bottom line in this case, as in many similar situations, is that you respected your body by attempting to remedy the dissonance, and you planted a seed of awareness for the other person to recognize in the future!

The dissonance of war

Your body is extremely sensitive to situations that pose an ever present possibility that you would have to destroy somebody or even be involved indirectly in the destruction of another person or the witnessing of trauma inflicted on innocent people. No matter how much you may think you "like" the strategic aspects and aggressive physicality of combat and believe that you can handle it, when your body is placed in the negative energy of a war zone, it is one of the deepest pins that your body can be exposed to. You *will* be stressed-in! Just ask the estimated 300,000 of those U.S. troops placed in Iraq or Afghanistan, who have been labeled with PTSD and are struggling to find the keys to heal their neighborhood so as to quiet their anxiety and depression symptoms!

From an early age, we are exposed to war and violence "from a distance" via cartoons, television, movies, and certain spectator sports. From a distance we don't overtly feel the impact, but our bodies are still buffering strongly. When we directly involve our bodies at the next level, such as when the youngster handles toy soldiers and guns, pretending to kill, but especially video games where we are now pushing buttons to kill, the body buffering is even more profound.

You can argue all you want, but your body and spirit do not resonate at all with the energy of warfare or violence. The compassion inside you kicks in when somebody really gets hurt…then you feel it…don't you? For example, your mind makes you think you like the fight at the game, but if someone ends up lying on the ground or ice, motionless or bleeding, you get quiet and concerned, don't you? Your body feels different. That being said, I will repeat that the energy of war is a dissonance that will stress in every participant, whether you immediately recognize it or not! The dissonance of war squeezes your body so hard, because *your body wants you out of there,* and maximally healthy focus is your best chance.

Did you know that your neighborhood has a campus? It's called the hippocampus. It's not too far from your neighborhood hypothalamus. The dissonance of war is so tough on your neighborhood that it actually can stress-in your campus! Your hippocampus is involved with memory...thus, not a pretty picture to disrupt its harmony, because you need the ability to generate an abundance of good memories to relegate the imprinted dissonance of war memories to the sidelines. In fact, all the sections of your neighborhood with the unusual names – hypothalamus, hippocampus and, amygdala – are squeezed hard. The lingering effects of the dissonance of war are well known. The keys to loosening this deep pin are found within this text, especially in the discussions of emotional energy management and the higher influences.

A word about dissonance and phobias: There is a fine line between temporary situational symptoms of dissonance that are on the normal bell curve, and what healthcare professionals would call a phobia. For example, it is *not* phobic for your body to feel very uncomfortable riding in or getting stuck in a cramped, old, dimly lit, under-ventilated elevator in an old building. It is very acutely dissonant for many people and symptoms are not unexpected. Our body was not meant to ignore the energy of being trapped in a small space such as this elevator or a closet...it is oppressive. Many of the same people are just fine in a large, well-lit elevator that may or may not have a clear glass side to look out of. In the same vein, it is within our body's normal response not to necessarily enjoy dangling at the top of an amusement park ride or walking near the edge of a cliff. You get the picture.

How many of you classify yourself as having a phobia to injections (needles)? Well, many of you can declassify yourselves, because the anticipation of having an unnatural energy forcefully injected under your skin with a sharp object is dissonant to the human body, 100% of the time, whether or not you get obvious symptoms. How about air travel? This is double body dissonance – the dissonance of heights and tight spaces! No*body* is at ease on an airplane. Your body is never refreshed after a flight. In addition, as you now understand, all air travel subjects your body to the stress-in effects related to an altered status quo with gravity and cosmic radiation.

Now, if you do actually insert fear, then subtle symptoms may become intensely dramatic (such as profuse sweating, fainting, etc.). Persistently inserting truly phobic shades of fear will chronically stress you in, and your emotional brain (hypothalamus, amygdala, etc.) is once again at center stage. You have heard the unfortunate phrase "familiarity breeds contempt"? Well, to confront phobias within the *natural* spectrum (living organisms, natural events), you must understand that familiarity (with what you fear) breeds *respect,* which, in turn, can significantly reduce your tendency to insert fear. In other words, acquire as much knowledge as you can about nature's *purpose* for that which you fear.

Here is a true example of this: Many of you may have been aware of the struggles of the honey bee population in recent years. One gentleman who would startle rather easily around bees took an interest in the bees' plight and began to research this story. Prior to this time, if a bee ever landed on his clothes or buzzed by, his startle was rather dramatic. He decided to write a short article about the bees and their incredible contribution to our natural produce supply. If he noticed a bee on the ground that had died, he would pick it up and place it on the grass. Then a very interesting thing happened one day. He was sitting out in the yard reading a book when a bee flew onto his pant leg. He did not startle, nor was there even a hint of tenseness of his muscles!

Now, does this mean that if you research snakes or spiders you won't startle if you see one near? Not necessarily, but understanding their role in the order of nature and respecting their natural boundaries will significantly decrease the chance that a snake or spider will ever harm you.

Should you fear lightning? No, but you should know what its purpose is (yes, lightning is a purposeful natural event) and respect its boundaries by not going out to hit golf balls with your irons during a thundershower. What about microorganisms… what we have labeled as "germs"? We have more microorganisms within our body space than we have cells. Since fear stresses you in, it will affect your immune system. So, fear of a microorganism getting by your neighborhood defenses makes it more likely that it will. Every microorganism can cause dis-ease because all microorganisms are opportunistic. In other words, every one (even the "helpful" bacteria within our digestive tract) will take the opportunity to "explore" if given the chance. Stress energy and disrespectful actions give them the chance. Many of the most "feared" microorganisms that had their own secluded place in nature were able to "jump ship" due to the following:

1) indiscriminate and disrespectful animal farming and consumption;

2) indiscriminate and disrespectful use of antibiotics and disinfectants; and

3) indiscriminate and disrespectful body-to-body contact.

Thus, we do not, and may never, know what initial purpose these mysterious bits of energy had because we didn't respect their boundaries and now they have mutated and propagated beyond what Nature intended! The bottom line: **Fear punches**

holes in your immune system. Disrespectful acts ambush your immune system. Therefore, stay balanced, using all the natural and healthy keys within the text and use healthy focus to make respectful decisions!

Here are some mind-awakening joules for thought. If you look back in history you will find that many documented infectious epidemics and pandemics have occurred in relation to the following: 1) During the time of war and its profoundly negative ambient energy (the pandemic of 1918, for example, that occurred after four years of world war and killed more people than the war battles themselves!); 2) during times of indiscriminate urbanization/colonization without regard for proper sanitation; and 3) during times of migration of people, including people who were fleeing from oppressive energy.

So where do we stand now? Well, come to think of it, in the past 70 years we have continued with war after war; we now have indiscriminate deforestation without regard for natural compensation, and we have more people on the move regionally and worldwide…large numbers feeling isolated and unsettled due to fear and oppression. The ambient energies of these actions stress all of us in. Please remind yourself that the bonds of the staircase are being strained and branches of the tree are struggling to thrive. If the staircase unravels or if enough branches disconnect from their natural roots, your neighborhood will be devastated regardless of where you are or what you possess. Beautiful minds working together can find healthy solutions to our global crisis!

CHAPTER SEVEN

GOOD VIBRATIONS

Your emotional brain certainly will appreciate your releasing the stuffed emotions and removing all the "pins" of the unresolved and dissonant energies so that its thermostat can run smoothly. However, it also requires waves of good vibrations to maintain a good natural flow and balance of our "feel good" neuropeptides to our entire body. In the physical realm, here are specific examples of what can really help:

Smiles and laughter

These encourage the release of healing neuropeptides and can positively affect your immune system. Consider a true naturally formed smile to be a loving wink from your body and soul, especially in response to good energy. With our capacity to harbor a beautiful mind, we can also choose to present a smile to others even if it is a brief encounter with an unfamiliar face or a person who has been a challenge or a constant source of frustration. This can temporarily soften the inflexible and struggling mind of another. Consider natural laughter to be our body's release valve when we experience or reflect on life's truly spontaneous and benignly awkward moments.

Isn't it amazing how many different ways our body helps to make our paths easier? In contrast, if you find that you are smiling or laughing to belittle or to applaud another's misfortune, then it is generated from a struggling mind laced with varying degrees of anger, greed, and jealousy, and, yes, there is work to be done to beautify your mind.

Pleasant aromas

Did you know that nobody alive today has ever taken a breath of fresh air? The industrial revolution took care of that. As long as we continue to refine, burn, and spray, your body will not be able to experience fresh air no matter where you are on the planet. We get a glimpse of Heaven scent on Earth after a rain shower, when the air is briefly cleansed and nature's aromatherapeutic oils are released from the soil and foliage. This is invigorating and soothing at the same time. So, as has been said, take time to smell the roses and all of nature's finest – especially natural foliage, flowers, spices, organic fruits, and vegetables. If your everyday working environment does not support a variety of natural fragrances and/or your air quality is very suboptimal, bring some plant life into your dwelling space, as natural foliage helps to refresh and detoxify your air as well as offering a variety of aromas.

Music

Music = good sound vibrations = very positive energy. You never want to use the word "bad" with music. There is music and there is noise. It's time for the world to accept this concise definition. The word "music" demands this respect, since it really is the "universe-all" language. Noise, as you have already learned, is dissonant and stresses us in. You already know life is all about vibration, and music is a healing energy.

Music is not confined to instruments…it is any healing sound, such as the "music of the ocean waves." The study of sound vibration and its physiologic effect on the body is expanding and gaining traction. We already know that music can vibrate our emotional brain to healthy states of relaxation, euphoria, and invigoration. We have all experienced goose bumps and tears from music. (Your neighborhood hypothalamus is involved again!) Sometimes music may be the encouragement we need to get moving! Adult brains are more malleable than once thought, so music can produce some favorable connections within the brain at any age. In the case of children, it is becoming clear that music can encourage healthy focus for more efficient learning.

So, where is the fine line between noise and music? That, my friends, is the 64,000 joule question. Well, you can go the long route and wait decades for research to sort this out, or you can strive for a pristine neighborhood and find out rather soon. This includes listening to sound without the addition of any brain-altering substance. Your body will then clearly tell you what is music and what is noise. You will feel it.

Presently, many people use the extremes of sound as an attempt to soothe their emotional brain. For example, some use the most meditative sounds to drown out the fear and clutter in their minds, temporarily quieting their anxiety symptoms. Others use the most "heavy" sounds as a remedy for their boredom or depression symptoms. This use of sound may be temporarily helpful, but it does not release suppressed emotional energy or dissolve worry and fear. If you use the knowledge that is presented in the text, you will find that the most meditative music will be healing rather than a band-aid, and the most invigorating music will naturally enhance your feel good neuropeptides!

Esoteric "sound" for thought: When a piece of music is used to promote people, products, or deeds of questionable integrity, the imprint will be left on the music and will dampen its positive effect. This applies for words as well as visual effects associated with music. Therefore, be sure to screen out obvious toxic baggage when you listen to music! Here is a common example: television commercials. Almost all are looking to promote something, and adding music gives them some "feel good" energy. People in advertising know that the link becomes a permanent resident of your (hippo)campus. How many jingles do you know from childhood connected to food or toys? What good purpose have they served? Oftentimes, fragments or short musical phrases within a jingle are found within other musical compositions. How can you remember them word for word, note for note from so long ago? How many times have you found yourself humming a tune which then links to a tune of irrelevance?

Here's some news about your neighborhood campus: Repetitive exposures become high profile residents of your campus and are not leaving anytime soon. Our brains can store more detail than you may think. You do not need intruding linkage that is distorting the picture your neighborhood is trying to paint for you.

The bottom line: The natural flavor of nature's energy is what is truly healing! An apple is an apple, a rose is a rose, a cloud is a cloud, and music is music. There are many varieties of all of these, but the natural untainted flavor is the best energy. Thus, a waxed, chemically exposed apple is not an optimally healing flavor. A cloud shrouded in smog and contrails is not an optimally healing visual flavor, and music with certain added "bells and whistles" is not an optimally healing auditory flavor. And about those commercials, screen them, mute 'em, or boot 'em to keep your campus clean and green!

Loving touch

The largest organ of our body of force is our skin. It has sensors for infrared, pain, pressure, and even *vibration*. Our body needs human contact, electron-to-electron, force field-to-force field. Do not underestimate the importance of this. I am not talking about reproductive sexual energy. I'm talking about touch by someone who emits truly loving energy as being extremely healing. Babies cannot thrive without this. You know how wonderful your body feels during a skin-to-skin back rub or massage. A lot is going on within your body and emotional brain during those times. A lack of loving touch can lead to or worsen a "deficiency" of core healing energy, and must not be overlooked when evaluating someone with developing depression symptoms.

Hugs are especially important. Remember what a hug represents energetically. A hug is a gesture of unconditional love. It is your heart and soul that is acknowledging the other person's heart and soul. As you know, body and spirit are all good and all loving energy. It is not an acknowledgment that you love their mind, so be careful not to withhold hugs just because the person has been a challenge or source of frustration for you! For example, when your spouse or partner is struggling with a dissonant mind and you are just about treading water trying to deal with all the lean-spirited energy, it is often the case that you lose the desire for more intimate physical touch with that person. This is because in a more time-bonded relationship it is the beauty of the mind that reflects one's outward attractiveness energetically, and your body just cannot ignore that field of dissonance. However, even during a relation-drift, it is a healing gesture to offer a hug!

Therapeutic touch can extend beyond the human realm. For example, most people enjoy patting a dog or cat on the head, rubbing its neck or stroking its fur. This is actually therapeutic for you. A pet may even be life-supporting in regards to the more dependent among us, such as certain elderly populations and those with more serious body dis-ease. However, a pet is not a substitute for human loving touch, nor is it appropriate to acquire a pet to avoid dealing with your fears or suppressed emotions.

As one example, suppose your spouse brings a pet home one day, without ever having discussed it with you. This is a red flag. It is very unfair, especially if there are children saying, "Can we keep it? Can we keep it?" because it puts you on the spot. This animal, especially a dog, is going to be like another child, and taking care of its many needs will be chores (not positive vibes) for you, no matter how you try to convince yourself otherwise. Your spouse's action may be the sign of a relation-drift. Even if you are going to keep the pet, you need to have an honest dialogue to find out the *real* reason for this action. You may discover there are other issues that need to be brought to light.

Healthy sleep, healthy sleep, healthy sleep!

Physiologically, your neighborhood is equipped with a complex biological clock that prepares your body to relax so that your brain can focus on generating the healing and recharging waves of sleep. This occurs most naturally as daylight fades to nightfall – hence, the term "a good night's sleep." Since your brain is hanging out its "do not disturb" sign for one-quarter to one-third of your life's hours, you know how important this time is. So please be sure to honor its request. Your sleeping space must be uncluttered, quiet, air temperature comfortable, and naturally dark. Remember to keep your dwelling's wireless waves to a minimum and keep your head away from electromagnetic fields such as clocks and other "live" wires. Sleeping pills are band-aids that will stress you in when used chronically. If you commit to dealing with the root of your insomnia you will be able to release the sleep aid habit. Your body will love you for it.

CHAPTER EIGHT

SPIRITUAL INFLUENCES

The creative essence of the universe and not-so-subtle guiding energy

Events that people from all walks of life describe as beyond the realm of coincidence are too numerous to count and clearly reflect a universe that has its own guiding and creative essence. Remember that there is no chance, luck, or coincidence within the fabric of the natural universe. So, how do we continue with the theme of the text regarding body and energy when it comes to these esoteric "energies" and indescribable influences? We must go back to the one equation that you are now all familiar with. That is $e = mc^2$. Did you know that there is literally another side to this equation? The complete equation is as follows:

0 (vast space devoid of natural energy) $*=*$ $e = mc^2$.

Do you see it? Where did all of the e (natural energy of the entire universe) come from? If there was a big bang, what filled the tiny bubble of space with all the energy of the universe before the expansion? Where did that energy come from? You can go on to infinity, and still there had to be a primary catalyst, *=*, which was creative. This scientifically unsolvable equation is what shatters the boundaries of physics and allows us to enter the dimensions of spirituality.

Let's talk facts. The overwhelming majority of people in the world, most likely you also, believe in a Divine influence…a creative essence. Most refer to this influence as God, many as Source. The fact is, we can't further classify the Divine as an energy, force or otherwise, because we are not privy to that knowledge. However, every *body* literally contains sparks of this indescribable, infinite, creative essence and, thus, everybody has the potential to consciously experience an ever deepening connection to the highest essence. How do we begin to describe the seemingly indescribable?

There are two other influences that also cannot be classified and are the most healing influences we experience. They are Love and Knowledge.

Let's begin with love. You will not find an equation or particle that captures its essence. Yes, we can clearly feel the effects of love and see how our own neighborhood responds energetically to this influence. Love itself, however, resides within the higher influences. I guarantee that there is not one person reading this text who wouldn't agree that a loving influence places their body in a unique and unparalleled state of ease.

Here is a true account that speaks volumes about love. A person experiencing chronic "unexplained" symptoms of pain had a mind full of fear, guilt, and anger, but clearly described having a wonderful sense of ease and pain-free state when exposed to loving kindness. This person would frequently say, "If I could be showered with a fire hose of love, I would feel wonderful."

These were the exact words. This is one example which confirms that the loving influence can immediately soothe the mind and even transmute the negative energetic influences of fear, anger and guilt. Of course, for a sustained state of ease, this person must choose to release the negative mind energies and reconnect to the loving influences of her inner light and the highest essence.

Is it possible that Love can actually *dissolve* these negative energetic influences? An influence that can dissolve energy is supposed to be an unsolvable equation because energy can be transformed, but not erased. How can this be? Remember the other side of the equation? Only a higher influence can catalyze negative energies back to nothingness! It's beautiful, isn't it? How many of you have "goose bumps" right now reading this?

Knowledge as a higher influence may seem like more of a challenge for you to grasp, but it really isn't. You may argue that knowledge is energetic imprinting in your campus. This is not accurate. It is *information* that is energetically imprinted within your neighborhood campus. Remember how we discussed mankind-generated wireless waves. They all send information… not knowledge. The Internet is described as the information superhighway, not the knowledge superhighway! There are many people who have a lot of information that packs their campus, but have not added to their original foundation of knowledge.

Knowledge is the understanding of what everything represents energetically, in other words, the meaning. Since only the creator of something can know what the exact meaning of the creation is, and all the elemental building blocks in our universe trace back to a higher influence, then knowledge…like love…is in a class of very Divine company. As humans, even though we are still in the seedling stage when it comes to the deepest Knowledge, we are reaching a critical level of collective knowledge that can tip the balance in favor of Health on Earth. Can you imagine what it would be like if we knew exactly what everything represented energetically? Although we cannot know everything, you now have a primer within this text to strengthen your foundation of knowledge. Can knowledge dissolve or transmute fear, guilt, and anger? Yes.

To reinforce your understanding of the higher levels of love and knowledge, ask yourself, what can never be taken from you? Love and knowledge, and of course, faith in a higher influence. Thus, God is the essence of Love and Knowledge. Your spirit holds your connection to purpose. The most purposeful and ultimately healing gifts you can give to anybody are love and knowledge. Your children will become incredibly healthy and aware if they are showered with these influences from an early age. I guarantee it.

You may be familiar with the quote, "Coincidence is God's way of remaining anonymous." On first thought, it appears to be a clever and insightful phrase. However, it is very far from the truth. God is clearly not in the realm of anonymity. To the contrary, God is the epitome of omnipresence. One of God's manifestations is called synchronicity (not coincidence). Synchronicity serves as an eye-opening, mind-awakening reminder that there are natural energies and higher influences that can actually steer you in a purposeful direction. If you have any thoughts about debating the existence of a universal guidance, you should take a deep breath and awaken, because you already know that your quarks and electrons, and especially your good friend Gravity, all have attractive properties and are guiding in their own way. There is guiding synchronicity and creative synchronicity. How they will affect your body is totally dependent on the nature of ***your*** thoughts and actions.

Did you know that your quarks and electrons may be shaped like strings? Physicists are still working on the math, but it is a most intriguing and viable model. Visualizing your neighborhood as vibrating strings will make it easier for you to picture the reality of resonance, synchronicity, and traction within the fabric of the universe and how it relates to your body!

We will first look at guiding synchronicity, which I describe as the *epinatural* energy of the universe. I use the term "epinatural" because of the parallels to the epigenome. As you now know, your epigenome fine tunes your DNA strings as you beautify your mind and come more into alignment within the natural fabric. Likewise, the guiding energy of the universe naturally vibrates your body strings, in turn guiding your body towards connections that resonate with your *good purposeful thoughts!* In essence, it is nature's way of truly pulling strings for you.

However, there is one catch. To get traction with your body, the energy generated by your mind must resonate with the epinatural! Fear, anger, guilt, and especially the ungenerous mind (a mind with greed, jealousy, possessiveness or stinginess), are major barriers to this connection. Since there are no universal frequencies that resonate with these negative energetic influences, the epinatural energies lose traction with your strings as you choose to generate a cloud of dissonance around you. Thus, it is not that the epinatural energy pulls away from you, it is the fact that you are pulling yourself out of the loop! You are making yourself scarce – disappearing from view, so to speak. As long as you choose dissonant thoughts (especially in the ungenerous category) as your guide, there will be less guiding synchronicity in your favor, and, no matter how large a quantity of material possessions you acquire, you will not be able to connect the dots that lead to a truly purposeful and joyous life.

Creative synchronicity moves directly from the realm of the higher influences. A highest essence can help us in an infinite number of ways. Since we have free will, what would a highest creative essence that is equal to Love plus Knowledge want to do for us to bring good thoughts to light? That would be to create energy that will cultivate a good purposeful thought once one *commits* to set it in motion. A good purposeful thought or idea that takes shape and manifests is one that always leads to more love and knowledge for people and ultimately to a higher level of health!

The key to creative synchronicity is commitment or movement. As many have said over the centuries, "The moment one commits oneself, then Providence moves too."

So, you ask, what happens if you take a negative energetic thought and put it in motion? Well, my friends, that is one of the most disrespectful actions you can perform in the light of your life Source. In other words, when you take waves of anger, fear, greed, jealousy, and possessiveness and put them into motion through violence, oppression, stinginess and intimidation, you are hindering another's capacity to work their passion, find their purpose, and contribute their gifts to humanity. This is a heavy energetic blow to *your* body, because *you* are choosing to distance yourself from Love. **It is not possible to realize a life even remotely close to your highest and best potential without a strong connection to Love. This is the one ingredient that brings everything into alignment.**

Since no viable relationship is one-sided, and the highest essence is Love, then how do we love Love? The answer is not speculative. It is evidence-based throughout history and into the present. First, you must acknowledge that your interactive environment is the entire universe. You now know this to be the truth.

Second, you need to **open a line of mindful communication** by sending some thought energy into this space without boundaries. Most of you would think of this as prayer. When you recite loving passages from divinely inspired scripture, it is certainly good energy-in-motion. However, it is vitally important that you also **dialogue in your own way by asking questions!** Specifically, do this by using thought energy or spoken words to ask for an understanding to come through regarding a life challenge or to further your knowledge of nature's good fabric so that you can apply this understanding (knowledge) for your best life ongoing and for the greater good. In essence…ask for guidance! You must be patient. We do not know the timing of when the understanding will come through. As I like to say, "Just leave a sincere and purposeful message on the universe's answering machine and the highest essence will respond in kind." Remember, your own sincere spontaneous request for understanding is vital for your life and ongoing health.

Third, you love a creative essence by respecting the natural essence of what has been created. By this I mean, beautifying your mind, balancing yourself with all of nature's energies to keep your neighborhood pristine, and showering others with love, whether through communication with passion to awaken the sleeper, or by sharing pure love and knowledge.

Always remember that **Love will never stop loving you.** A lack of synchronicity or healing emotions only occurs when *you* choose to distance yourself from Love. If you refuse to trust in a highest essence or choose to consistently display actions that are ungenerous, hindering, or destructive, you will always experience at least some degree of depression symptoms, which is your body literally crying out for you to tune back in to Love.

Thus, be sure to maintain a sincere and steady dialogue. After all, there is an infinite amount of love and knowledge that can be acquired from a Source that is Love and Knowledge itself. Unfortunately, many of you only "make the call" during a major challenge. When you wait until a major challenge to make the call, your mind sees challenge as crisis and you will almost always insert fear.

Here is a simple metaphorical description of this. Suppose you are walking the path of life and, as we all have experienced from time to time, an especially challenging life situation develops. The visibility becomes very poor along the path and you do not know what to do. Wouldn't it be great if "transportation" came by to get you through the fog? If you already have an open line of communication with the creative essence, this vehicle will be there instantaneously. How far you will be guided will depend on how courageous you are in trusting the path of the vehicle as you travel along new paths.

Isn't it interesting that many people only "make the call" when faced with a potential life or physical death situation (a heart attack, lost at sea, etc.), suddenly looking up to the sky and pleading with the highest essence (you pray) to please help you? Since a Loving creative essence is not only all powerful, but also all benevolent, this essence will still show up to contribute understanding to the situation whatever the outcome, because at least you acknowledged the existence of this essence by starting a dialogue! What is unfortunate is that as soon as you are out of the woods, so to speak, many of you no longer maintain a dialogue.

Gratitude, respect, and benevolence are infinitely powerful influences that will allow your communication with the universe to be clear and strong. The depth of their influence on humanity is profound. You must never use the word "lovesick" or the term "unlucky in love," as the words "sick" and "unlucky" have no meaning in the context of the universe, and **Love is the essence of meaning.**

CHAPTER NINE

RELEASING STRINGS

One of the most important aspects of the universal energy spectrum is related to *release*. From this point on, you should no longer use the phrase "burning bridges," because it is inaccurate and obsolete. As you are now becoming an expert in understanding the energetic nature of the universe, you know that there are no bridges between people. We are all part of a fabric of energy where connections are instantaneous and ever present. You can't burn something that isn't there, and you can't keep a person's energy from engaging you.

The advice, you can't burn that bridge, comes from, and generates, a dissonance of fear and greed. It basically encourages you not to be yourself and to suppress your emotions because another person may be able keep you in "the game" that society and governments have convinced us we have to play. In plain terms, the mindset is, you decide that you can't say anything to a particular person because they are "connected" and may be able to do something for you someday. The rules of this game require you to dim your shining star, suppress your true emotions by not saying how you really feel, learn to attain positions of responsibility without having the credentials, and view everyone as your competitor. All of this is to possibly gain monetary and material resources, which we are led to believe will make us happy and healthy. *You do not have to do any of this.* In fact, that game is toxic and has stressed in every person who has ever played.

Many of you may remember the movie where a government computer starts to play a simulated game of global thermonuclear war. When the simulated bombs from all directions hit the U.S., the computer began to search for the launch codes to actually launch real missiles. The insightful young man in the control room finds a basic program of tic-tac-toe that the computer engages. He places it on auto play so that the computer plays itself. The computer plays faster and faster but every game ends in a tie. The computer eventually overheats and then comes back online. It has voice capability and says, "Good evening, professor…….. interesting game…….the only winning move is not to play."

The only winning move is not to play!

Here is what happens when you choose to play this game. Many of you seek to form bonds based on "If you scratch my back, I'll scratch yours." Every one of these attachments is a thread that's foreign to the natural fabric of the universe. Others keep count of times that you have "helped" someone, saying to the other person, "You owe me one." You keep score and expect an equal amount of "favors in return." This weaves more threads into your new web. Third, some of you may actively seek favors from others to circumvent the normal flow of life by "pulling strings" so you can attain a position you would not have had otherwise. This adds to your web. The problem is, you have spun a web *outside* of the natural fabric and are using it as your guide. In essence, you are disrespecting the universe and the creative essence, and you will ultimately end up in a place where you feel "lost" and unfulfilled. This is not speculation.

Most of you know of a song that arguably may be the world's most recognized tune composed by the most recognized band in history. You may not like the grammar, but a line goes "Nowhere you can be that isn't where you are meant to be."

Simple, yet profound. Please be sure you remember this. By the way, the song just happens to be specifically about love and the word "love" is spoken almost one hundred times during this song. It simply relates the truth. That is, if you strive to align ever more completely within the natural fabric (Love), you will always be where you are supposed to be for your best life.

Another line in the song goes, "Nothing you can know that isn't known." Beautiful, isn't it? This is another reference that reflects on the fact that all knowledge is already out there for us. We just have to acquire it as we move within the fabric. You will not find it on your self-spun web! So we are back to love and knowledge again. If you insist on using the metaphor of a "game of life," then please play within the correct game! Play the most healthy game, where your good thoughts and actions allow synchronicity to guide the pieces on the game board and where everybody wins as they are able to work their passion with purpose!

Thus, to begin to release strings and unravel the web, you must do the following: throw away any score cards your mind is holding. The past is past. Allow the future to evolve and respond to situations as they arise. It is most important to remember that whenever you help someone, do it without any expectation of receiving any "favors" in return. Helping another with good purpose also helps you energetically, as you now know. Don't actively seek people to "pull strings" for you or a dependent to circumvent a natural process. If synchronicity brings someone into your space, that is meant to be.

I want to clarify the balance involved with helping someone. Remember that a beautiful mind can navigate the line between selfless and self-first without ever being selfish. This means that as you find a situation where you are in an opportune position to help someone with purpose, be sure that you can do so within your means. The energies must balance. For example, if you volunteer to help others for so many hours that you sacrifice healthy sleep, nutrition, and personal time with your dependents, your body will suffer and you will ultimately have less energy to help others. Remember, even helping one person with good purpose initiates an infinite chain of positive energy!

There are many other life examples where release is therapeutic. Not just putting the cart before the horse, but actually releasing the cart from the horse. For example, how many of you become aware, even "painfully" aware, that your body is not at ease within your current work/job activities, and you wonder how you can find a way to use your unique and special gifts to work your passion with good purpose? Since most governments and societies have not been structured to reward people for having the courage to transition to a more inspiring and fulfilling career, it is easy to insert fear and choose to tolerate the position you are in. This always stresses you in and often manifests as obvious dis-ease. Since many of you may be in this boat, how does one identify what their unique niche is? That is another 64,000 joule question. The answer is closer than you think.

Here's the thought process to get you moving in a good "direction" to find a passion that you can work with good purpose. Take some time in your favorite quiet uncluttered space to reflect. There are three things to keep in mind when looking for this answer.

First: Completely remove money from the equation. Money is not a guiding energy. It is a red herring when it comes to guidance. In fact, it may be the red herring of all red herrings (a topic for another place and time). For those who are not familiar with the term "red herring," it is a metaphor for something that distracts you from the true issues at hand, and when used as guidance, it leads nowhere! Thus, forging your career based on following the trail of money will ultimately leave you unfulfilled. This specific energetic imbalance will often lead to symptoms of depression.

Second: Write down everything that comes easily to you; everything that you love to do; and everything that really piques your interest for more knowledge.

Third: Highlight everything on the list that could create the opportunity for you to *help other people* realize their highest and naturally best potential. The word "realize" is not a synonym for purchase! Get the drift? Now, generate an abundance of reflective thought energy and dedicated research towards these highlighted areas, with the primary goal of empowering others, and you will experience synchronicity at its best as your vision takes shape.

CHAPTER TEN

THE VIBRATION OF DESIRE

How does one describe the vibration that moves us to natural intimacy? Some call it a drive...some say desire...some even refer to it as a symptom. However you frame it, this vibration is in place to enable conception. You can philosophize all you want, but that is its core purpose. It's a powerful vibe. It has to be, considering that the natural continuum of humanity is dependent on it.

As we have discussed in previous chapters, the body, for our benefit, is resolutely consistent in its ways and does not take time to debate or ponder its natural obligations. So it should be no surprise that naturally intimate body contact between a fertile man and woman *can* result in a new body being conceived regardless of any attempt to otherwise prevent it. This is well documented. As long as there is a viable ovary and one spermatozoon, there is always the possibility that the neighborhood will find a way, even in the most unlikely of circumstances.

Although this vibe/natural conceptive intimacy connection is quite obvious, the importance of what happens between vibe and consent has been literally lost in translation. In other words, societal and cultural influences have generated enough of a smokescreen of indifference and misinformation to keep our physically maturing children in the dark regarding the virtues of patience and the truth about loving relationships. Multimedia has certainly generated enough audio-visual waves to influence our younger generation to believe that intimacy is equivalent to love or that engaging in intimacy is a prerequisite for establishing a meaningful loving bond. This could not be further from the truth, although your children's peers may try to convince them otherwise.

Recall how the unsettled mind can distort one's body guidance. Even regarding this vibe and other seemingly unmistakable body guidance, the unsettled mind can lead us astray.

For example, the vibration of hunger is a body guidance, but there are many people who admit that they chronically find themselves eating (e.g., sweets), thinking that their body was guiding them to consume food, when in fact this was not the case. They admit that, aside from the momentary "fix", the action did not result in ease. Many come to recognize the fact that these "urges" seem to peak at times when they insert worry and experience anxiety symptoms. This represents a mind of chronically inserted fear retracing an old familiar path, looking for a temporary band-aid of comfort.

In the same vein, people often act on the urge to release energy sexually, in an attempt to soothe their anxiety or depression symptoms, without recognizing that it is a mind's red herring. Many discover the truth of this, i.e., they awaken to the fact that they have been "looking for love in all the wrong places."

At this point on humanity's learning curve of awareness, children, as they physically mature into young adults, always lag behind emotionally and spiritually. This maturity gap can, and will, narrow significantly when we, as parents, guardians, educators and other prominent influences in children's lives, become in-sync and on the same page with each other regarding the naturally best anticipatory guidance from very early on.

Since our efforts to instill the virtues of patience and adult-level responsibility have not produced a sustained ripple of influence, as evidenced by the continued pandemic of sexually acquired infection and post-conceptive controversy, what can we tell children, as they physically mature into fertile young adults, that will actually stay in their mind's eye? The answer, as always, begins with honest knowledge-based communication.

Before you begin this discussion with your child, be sure to communicate that you are not telling them what they can or cannot do. Explain that you are sharing knowledge about what a person's body naturally experiences as they become young adults, and what this physical maturation means in terms of adult relationships. You should mention that many older adults will admit that they would have very much appreciated having had this knowledge shared with them when they were your child's age.

If you still get the "I already know the facts about sex, so we really do not have to have this discussion," please share a story such as the following:

> "When you were very young, you were playing with a ball and it rolled into the street. You ran to get the ball without any knowledge that a motor vehicle could run you over. All you 'knew' was that the toy was fun and that if you didn't retrieve it you would be unhappy. I ran and picked you up before you ran into the street. Of course you were kicking, screaming and crying because you could not understand why I would keep you from your toy. You didn't know that my action was based on love and life-saving knowledge that I had and you did not. You are older now, but so am I. You will encounter similar situations, but at an adult level. Since you are

now a young adult with more space to navigate, I will not always be at your side if you choose to run after a moment of desire or passion without knowing the true consequences. Because I love you, I am picking you up now so that you do not get run over as you make your own choices."

This will get their attention.

Virtually every parent will have a situation similar to this one to share with the child. Even if you don't, you can still use this common, true life type of event to make the point. Children can grasp the meaning behind it.

Begin by affirming that your child's body is undergoing a physical hormonal awakening. This physical awakening naturally brings with it fertility and the vibe that leads us to natural intimacy. Point out that the alignment of these events is not by chance. The core purpose of the vibe and natural intimacy is to enable conception.

Is natural intimacy meant to be a part of mature adult loving human relationships? Yes, but it is not equivalent to love, nor a prerequisite or requirement for a loving relationship. Is natural intimacy meant to be naturally pleasurable? Yes, but it is not in place solely for a moment of pleasure, nor is it a release valve for their emotional stress energy. Children must also be aware that their peers may try to convince them that engaging in the naturally intimate "will represent a feather in their cap," or that consent "is necessary to 'win' the love of another." All of these are examples of consent to natural intimacy that is misaligned with its purpose.

You can explain, in your own words, the fact that a woman's fertile body, month after month with remarkable consistency, meticulously prepares the womb in anticipation of the conceived, and if conception occurs there is no other time where the body commits so much physiologically to accommodate a natural purpose. There is clearly nothing casual in the body's approach to the act of intimacy. Thus, it should be no surprise that any indiscriminate or casual approach that one takes with natural intimacy is misaligned, and brings with it an increased risk of acquiring opportunistic microorganisms. Have your child look up the national and worldwide incidence of sexually acquired infection (a.k.a. STD's) if they need further awakening.

Since the body is naturally conceptive, any mindset that is "contra-ceptive" is also misaligned. When one has a contra-ceptive mindset, this means that one is carrying at least some shade of fear regarding conception, pregnancy, and/or parenting. Fear, as you have learned, punches holes in your immune system.

In addition, fear of conception, of pregnancy, or of parenting brings with it an increased risk of fear-based decisions if conception occurs. Fear-based decisions bring an increased risk of guilt, even catastrophic guilt, and chronic depression symptoms, for the female as well as for the male partner. You should know that the degree to which misaligned consent leads to depression symptoms and the insertion of guilt has been grossly underestimated.

In the last half century, the idea of "intimacy solely for pleasure" has spawned the development and widespread use of hormone-based contraceptives (i.e., birth control pills, patches, et. al.), all of which stress-in the body and offer no protection against acquiring opportunistic microorganisms. Their use is also enabling to those who would not otherwise venture into the realm of indiscriminate and casual intimacy.

There seems to be a persistently prevalent mindset among young adults that involves the idea that natural intimacy must be practiced to become a mature loving partner. Your child will almost never bring this up, but it is almost always lurking somewhere in their mind. Please present the following newsflash: "No experience necessary!" The idea that natural intimacy is an audition for a spot in a mature loving partnership is an "urban myth." The fact is, and this is the icing on the cake of your discussion, patience is actually what needs to be practiced. Use it or lose it refers to patience, not natural intimacy. Patience, in the face of passion, is incredibly powerful in the natural universe and beyond. It brings with it synchronicity to encounter others who are more mature, and is a catalyst for a deeper understanding of love.

Highlight the fact that the ability to demonstrate patience in the face of passion is one major feature that distinguishes human beings from every other living organism. Patience is not suppressive, it is impressive! That is why consent to natural intimacy is most aligned within a committed relationship where both the female and the male partners have personally matured to the level of knowing that they will fulfill their natural maternal and paternal obligations, should conception occur. If a critical mass of our young adult children can be mindful of this and refrain from running into the path of a "streetcar named desire," a positive ripple of influence can be sustained. After all, if only one of the two partners is mature and aware enough to recognize when passion is misaligned, there will be no engagement in physical intimacy at that point in time. This may awaken the other to a more mature mindset.

Beyond the discussion with your child, there are joules for thought that you, as adults, must keep in mind. Patience is a loving influence. Only when people awaken to the fact that patience, in this regard, can be a catalyst for personal maturity and alignment with purpose, even for those in the most challenging of living conditions, will we see a return to a natural balance in the realm of the intimate.

Regarding conception itself, there also seems to be a void in knowledge regarding the very early childhood neighborhood. Assumptions and rationalizations abound when discussing the nature of our earliest days. Presently, belief, opinion and interpretation across the societal and cultural landscape are all over the map in regards to the timing of when consciousness begins. The short answer: "Only God knows." The long answer: Only God knows, and this is one reason why we may not: Most people have been led to believe that consciousness is the same as brainwaves. This is false. Brainwaves are a reflection of a facet of consciousness, but we have yet to understand the entire spectrum.

Take dreams, for example. We still do not know what they represent exactly. Yes, we can measure alterations in physiology reflecting a dream state, but we still cannot grasp its origins or be sure of a dream's meaning. Thus, brainwaves can reflect a facet of consciousness, but we cannot conclude that all consciousness is brainwaves.

Let's look at an example that illustrates the slippery slope of assumption and extrapolation. Water has subtle properties that we still do not fully understand. As warm water cools, it becomes more dense. Thus, you might extrapolate that it would continue to become more dense as it approaches freezing and beyond, to become ice. However, this is not the case. It becomes less dense!

The word "dense" is often used to describe someone who is not aware. It's often used in a lean-spirited context, but let's use it metaphorically in a greener context to illustrate a point. As adults, when our brains are more fully developed, we generally see ourselves as being less "dense" (i.e., more aware). Extrapolating back through childhood, as we see the brain smaller in size and the maturity level decreased, we would describe the earlier stages as progressively more dense (less aware). As we move to the very early fetus and embryo stages, we see a transition to where we no longer recognize a brain as we know it. However, how do you know that this stage is not *less* dense (i.e., more "aware")? It looks different, as ice looks different from water, but it is not necessarily less conscious!

There is one truth about our physical life that we do know with certainty. That is, from bookend to bookend of our physical existence we can always call ourselves a body. A body is defined as the contiguous physical structure at any point in time, and not by a specific number of cells or a required number of body parts. This is not in dispute, otherwise those of you who have had a gallbladder, spleen, appendix, or other organ removed would no longer be considered a body. We certainly do not label one who never manifests a complete set of ribs, vertebrae, or teeth an incomplete body. Thus, you can literally and figuratively consider your physical life to be a seamless "body of work," whether 8 cells or 8 trillion, from conception to the other bookend of passage.

Whatever you choose to believe regarding when consciousness begins, the fact is that conception results in a dynamic body of cells with its unique DNA vibration. Thus, in the new paradigm, you can also define a living human body as a unique collaboration of cells with the potential to harbor a beautiful mind. Regardless of our age or stage, doesn't this apply to all of us?

CHAPTER ELEVEN

BUILDING A SOLID FOUNDATION

Having moved from neutrinos and gravity, to photons, waves of humanity, and into the ultra-esoteric, I know that you may not have imagined how many visitors frequent your neighborhood on a 24/7 basis. Use the keys that have been presented, and you will attain your masters degree in bio-energy "wave" management. A crowning achievement! Your body will love you for it.

With so many visitors, you would think that there would be a lot of remodeling going on to keep your neighborhood strong and up-to-date. Actually, this is exactly what is happening. "New" quarks and electrons are coming in to replace others all the time. Your neighborhood is being remodeled 24/7 for the entirety of your physical life. Your body knows how to perfectly lay the brick and mortar. Your body even knows exactly how to extract and transport the natural building materials to the necessary places in your neighborhood. With all the inferior building materials "on (and in) the market" in this era of convenience foods, you need to be sure to select from the highest quality catalog: the catalog we know to contain "nature's finest."

For the building materials of your infrastructure, the body uses mostly fats, proteins, and minerals. Then we need the tools to keep your neighborhood well-maintained, such as vitamins and antioxidants. The highest quality materials and tools will allow your body to use your cleanest fuels, oxygen, and carbs, most efficiently.

All of these ingredients could not come together for health without one other vital ingredient. That would be water! Most of you may be aware that the majority of your neighborhood is water, so you can "thank" water for an abundance of your joules. Thus, as the water vibrates, given its abundance in your neighborhood, its energy is amplified relative to your entire body. So I would suggest that if you are going to tap your glasses together, to Divine words of good health, you do it with water and not alcohol (which is not a preventive care tool, as we will discuss later).

Now, let's simplify nutritional sustenance for you.

First: Any time that you refine, engineer, or process the foods of nature in any way, they become energetically inferior to the original.

Second: Any ingredient that is extracted from the foods of nature is energetically inferior to the original ingredient that was naturally bonded in the food.

Third: Any natural ingredient (vitamin or otherwise) that you attempt to copy and mass produce, even if it appears to be an exact chemical copy, is not the same energetically as the original.

Most important: Always think of nature's raw whole foods as a perfectly wrapped gift to your body! Here's how you can most easily grasp the physiology. Suppose you are eating an avocado.

This is a perfectly wrapped gift sliding by your tastebuds and into your neighborhood distribution center. When this gift arrives, your body's digestive tract knows exactly how to unwrap it, extract exactly what it needs, re-package these nutrients, and transport them to the exact destination that it is required. This process is very complex, but the metaphor is physiologically accurate. Among the many good energies within this avocado, we have many vitamins…a truly natural multivitamin.

When one attempts to equate this to a manufactured, extracted, or processed "uni-vitamin" or multivitamin, we encounter many problems. First, the gift wrapping is all wrong. A capsule or tablet, for example, is a package unfamiliar to the body, and its timing is always off. Then when the contents are released, there is a flood of detached vitamins (that is, removed from their natural context) which can jump your neighborhood's fences and gain access to your circulation without proper processing. Since the vibration is off-key, your body has to work with sub-quality tools, which will ultimately weaken your infrastructure.

The knowledgeable individuals in the medical community are now beginning to see the truth of this. Did you know that in most studies using vitamin supplements, the supplements have not fared much better than a placebo, and in some cases, the supplement group fared worse than the placebo group, with possible increased risks and side effects? What is very concerning is that these bits of unnaturally packaged energies may be feeding other pockets of already stressed-in cells in the body. Look up beta-carotene supplements/lung cancer in smokers, folic acid supplements/colon polyps, and vitamin supplements/prostate cancer cells.

Most of the wheat flour products available in the supermarket are sprinkled with detached vitamins! They call this enriched. In this case, rich may mean poor. How much disease and masking of symptoms has this caused for your body? What about vitamin "enriched" water? The beverage industry has put on a "full court press" via athletes and others to promote vitamin water. This beverage is not liquid enhancement. It is not respectful to the neighborhood. In addition to this, many organic products are now being instilled with detached vitamins. Please read labels! Therefore, never take a shotgun approach to vitamin supplements. Since there is no such thing as "health in a bottle" or "preventive care in a capsule" regarding vitamin or mineral supplements, please first have a solid and well-informed idea of why you are taking them.

The bottom line: You are allocating significant monetary resources to multivitamins, trace minerals, and even antioxidant extracts, based on your fear of possibly missing a key to healthy aging or because your body is presently not at ease. Thus, unless you have a specific extenuating medical circumstance or you are clearly manifesting an array of symptoms that can be *directly* attributed to a deficiency state which cannot be addressed through respectful lifestyle change, management of stress energy, or improved access to nature's complementary spectrum of whole foods, you are wasting your monetary resources and you are disrespecting your body.

One additional pearl: If you are a woman of childbearing age be sure to enjoy a daily salad of green leafy vegetables (such as lettuce or spinach) or other foods that contain natural vitamins, including vitamin B9 (folic acid), because by the time you may become aware of a missed menstruation, many days have passed since conception and your child's body requires early access to a supply of natural tools sufficient to lay its foundation, especially its core nervous system.

Oils

Let's return to nature's finest. This time, let's press the oil out and bottle it. Since bottled vegetable, fruit, and seed oils are so prevalent within our dietary habits and the topic of much debate, let's clarify what these fats represent. Since they are detached fats, they too can gain access to your neighborhood in quantities beyond that which your body desires. In addition, these detached fats continue to lose their good vibrations every moment that they are exposed to air, light, or heat.

Let's look at an oil that has been used for thousands of years and presently seems to be designated as the "healthy" oil. That would be olive oil. Most of you have been led to believe that bottled olive oil is naturally safe to use in generous amounts. This is false, as you now understand. Granted, if you can find a fresh, properly packaged virgin product, it is near the top of the list compared to other bottled oils. However, it is still not equivalent to nature's finest building materials. How many of you sop up generous amounts of olive oil at home or at a restaurant before you even begin your meal? Did you know that just three tablespoons of oil has over 40 grams of fat? This is almost 400 calories of pure fat presented unwrapped to your body. This is not good. In addition, any traces of anti-oxidants within the bottled oils are also detached and, thus, are of unclear benefit to the neighborhood. On the other hand, if you slice half an avocado and consume it with the bread or on the salad in lieu of the oil, you give a gift to your body of naturally packaged vitamins, minerals, fiber, protein, and natural fat. Did you know that the fat content of an entire avocado is less than the three tablespoons of oil? How about a dozen walnut halves to replace the oil? You get minerals, protein, and even a bonus of one type of omega-3 fat. Bottled flaxseed oil doesn't hold a candle, energetically, to a handful of fresh walnuts.

Thus, there are no bottled oils that are naturally better for you than nature's finest, but if you truly enjoy their flavor, please feel free to add sprinkles or drops of fresh, virgin, or unrefined and unheated oil that has not been extracted from a mankind genetically modified source, to complement the meal's taste. Your body can handle that.

Faux fats

If you take a detached fat and then factory-refine it, you get a product so energetically distant from the original that you must classify it as a faux fat. If you then force quarks and electrons to bond with this faux fat, a process called partial hydrogenation, the product is even worse. Most of the bottled oils that are on the shelves are refined. Most of the snack foods and bakery products with their relatively long shelf lives contain partially hydrogenated faux fats. Your body can't build properly with these fats. The widespread use of these "faux fats of convenience," including margarines and shortenings, over the past several decades has been a most significant factor contributing to lipid imbalances and arterial dis-ease. If you care about your body you must read labels. If a label lists partially hydrogenated or hydrogenated *anything*, do not buy it. If a bottled oil or spread does not say unrefined, virgin, or extra-virgin, do not buy it. See how quickly your choices can influence those in the food industry to awaken and rethink their goals.

Also, be aware that all significantly heated oils will leave at least some disruptive fats on whatever was cooking in it. Deep fried foods are an obvious example; also, significantly limit your consumption of the crispy, crunchy, salty snacks, such as chips, that have been baked or boiled in oil prior to packaging.

The bottom line:

Fats are not bad for you. You can't live without them. You need all natural fats including the saturated type. Just take steps to wean from the faux fats and replace them with real gifts to your body. Remember that refined is not "fine." If you have access to nature's finest, place raw unroasted nuts and seeds high on your list. Walnuts and almonds are good examples. Avocados are a unique oily fruit that is packed with nutrients. Of course, you must not forget that some of nature's marine inhabitants, such as salmon and sardines, are valuable sources of omega-3 fats. Be sure to consider only healthy sustainably wild-harvested varieties.

If you choose to consume meat and poultry, be aware that you can find a much more beneficial balance of fats, including omega 3's, if the animal has been permitted to graze naturally on grassy pastures.

Speaking of omega-3 fats, you may have noticed that this topic has been in the spotlight in recent years. There is a very good reason for the publicity. Compared to other fats, only a few grams can go a long way to assist your neighborhood, especially if you do not "drown" it with an overabundance of detached oils and faux fats.

This is especially important during pregnancy and as your child matures to adulthood, as the developing brain requires access to sufficient omega 3 fats to maintain its optimal integrity. However, be aware that, due to mining and industry, virtually all fish now have unnaturally high levels of displaced mercury, which is toxic to the brain. Thus, do your research to determine the safest and best animal and plant sources of omega-3's, whether from the land or sea.

I guarantee that if you make the effort to find a palatable status quo to improve the ratio between omega-3 and your other daily fats, your body will love you for it.

Protein

We have known for some time about the amino acid units the body uses for your neighborhood protein building blocks. Protein is more abundant across the natural food spectrum than you may have been led to believe. Thus, always keep in mind that your protein intake may be too heavily weighted on the meat and other animal product side, and it is possible that you are giving more protein to your neighborhood than it needs. You do not need detached protein supplements or supplemental neurotransmitters.

If you do consume meat or poultry, be aware that any benefit to your neighborhood is directly proportional to how well the animal was treated during its lifetime. If the animal was subjected to injections, unnatural feed, or unloving living conditions, this energy will be transferred to your body when consumed. It will stress you in. Thus, it behooves you to find out the farming source and how the animal was processed. Remember, products from animals permitted to graze naturally grassy pastures will be leaner and more energetically beneficial to your body.

No to GMO

There is another major storm on the horizon. This involves the question of safety of mankind genetically modified food. You will see this described as GMO. Mankind genetic engineering "edits" a plant's DNA strands by adding snippets of foreign DNA from other organisms. Science fiction…no, science fact and real disturbing, wouldn't you say? They say it is to strengthen the plant, but in reality it energetically weakens the integrity of the original and cripples its value as a good nutritional source! The modified plant can now manufacture proteins that are strange to its natural state and you consume them.

Remember, nature has held the patent on all forms of energy, including energy of nourishment, since the beginning of time. Nature performs its own natural modifications over time to stay in balance with its ecosystem. We cannot copy or improve on nature's patents. Any plant or other food source that is genetically engineered is energetically different from the original. Since its vibratory state is different, when it is ingested, it forces the body to either assimilate this foreign energy or work to usher it out of the neighborhood. Thus, by definition, mankind genetically modified foods always stress you in. Our sensitive immune system could certainly be very vulnerable to these influences, possibly manifesting as allergic symptoms or worse. How will you feel if you are the first to develop symptoms of a new dis-ease complex?

GMO soybeans and corn and their many byproducts have already infiltrated the food chain. You cannot compromise on this issue. If a product does not say organic or "no GMO", then any soy, corn, or other ingredients may well be GMO! Begin to wean yourself off of any unlabeled products. As we discussed with faux fats, see how fast the food industry awakens to rethinking their goals. You are respecting your body, and you are helping to awaken the sleeping corporate individuals who have forgotten that we are all branches of the same tree.

Be aware that government agencies have opened the door for products made from cloned animals to potentially be sold in food stores. This is another disaster waiting to take down your neighborhood. Please start the ball rolling on this issue also. If this happens where you live, tell your local food store that you will not buy their provisions unless they are labeled "not cloned." Then see how fast distributors label their meat products. Did you know that many foods are bombarded with waves "that really hurt" (remember X's and gammas?) as they are processed? What will be the next technological advance (or should I say "decline") to further denaturalize our food supply?

Calcium and Minerals

How many of you are confused about calcium, minerals, and your neighborhood bone health? If you are, you are not alone. After decades of research, even the most advanced scientists still do not have the equation that neatly ties everything together biochemically. The good news...you don't need to rely on any such equation to care for your bony skeleton! As always, if you use the natural keys, the blueprint is there for you. The reason for your confusion stems from the belief that you must worry about maintaining a certain bone density so that you won't fall and fracture something. That whole mindset is very negative and misleading. The first thing you must do is to ask the correct question! That is, how do I help my neighborhood keep my bony skeleton naturally balanced and strong?

What you need to understand is that less bone density doesn't mean that your bones are not strong! You are a unique individual, and there are many factors that determine bony strength beyond what a bone density x-ray film can tell you. So, when we ask the right question, we know that the following answers are *not* correct:

1) detached calcium and mineral supplements

2) animal milk calcium

3) prescription drugs

It's unfortunate that we are led to believe that these are our major options. In fact, they can all stress you in...especially the prescription drugs. You have already learned most of the keys as you have followed the text! So let's see the correct answers to the question of how to keep bones naturally strong.

1) Intelligent exercise! Yes, purposeful movement within the sea of gravity. The tug of vitality is crucial.

2) Sunny D! The sun hormone is on center stage when it comes to bone health.

3) Nature's spectrum of naturally wrapped minerals – many of the same foods that we discussed earlier, such as nuts, seeds, fruits, vegetables, and marine life. Yes, they have calcium.

4) Releasing suppressed emotions and addressing fear! Yes, this is very important. An *excess* of hormone (cortisol) that enters the neighborhood when the hypothalamus has to deal with an imbalance of emotional energy will affect the status quo within your skeleton. In fact, your hypothalamus has a multi-faceted role in bone health.

5) Avoidance of alcohol, tobacco smoke, and caffeine. All of these energies have the potential to alter the status quo between your bone balancing cells, osteoblasts and osteoclasts. In addition, some of you are especially sensitive to the unnatural effects that cola beverages (which are of no benefit to your neighborhood, anyway) and detached salt may have on your natural bony mass.

I know that some of you raised your eyebrows when you saw animal milk calcium on the "wrong answer" list, so let's discuss that. Whether or not we should consume animal dairy products has been the topic of heated debate for decades and will continue to be debated until the "cows come home." Pun intended. The core of the issue is whether it is natural to consume something that is meant to be consumed at the source (i.e., the nipple) by baby animals. On one hand, you may say that it is calcium that is naturally packaged, so our bodies should be able to process it reasonably well. However, if it is specifically meant for baby animals then it may not be naturally friendly to our body. Many people find that their body is not at ease with animal milk products, as they experience symptoms of respiratory dis-ease (e.g., congestion) and/or gastrointestinal dis-ease (bloating, cramps, etc.), to name a few.

In addition, most milk consumed by us is pasteurized (heated), sometimes skimmed of its fats, and usually has detached vitamins added before it is placed in its cartons or bottles – quite a departure from the original product. Thus, we cannot confirm that animal milk products can *naturally* contribute to bone strength.

Be aware that an abundance of natural resources are required to produce animal milk. Whatever you decide about this issue, make knowledgeable decisions for yourself and your dependents, and be very selective and mindful regarding the quantity and quality of dairy products. Stay within the organic realm as the energy is more optimal. And don't forget, just because they have small amounts of detached D added, dairy products do not in any way release you from the obligation to optimize your healthy sunny-D.

Carbs

By now you know that your neighborhood is sweet, in the sense of cool, but it doesn't want to be too sweet when it comes to fuel. That rhymes, doesn't it? It really does not like refined carbohydrates. Nature has a wide spectrum of foods to choose from that supply natural sugars and starches. It is really important to stay in the naturally gift-wrapped mode when you choose your carbs. As you have learned, refined (oil, grain, sugar, etc.) is not fine.

Enriched food products are not rich. And your neighborhood particularly does not enjoy high fructose corn syrup. If you like syrup, enjoy some pure maple syrup. If you like corn, eat an ear of non-GMO corn. If you want fructose, eat an apple. If you want a high, share your newfound knowledge with others! Helping others to help themselves is always a natural high! Also be aware that the more refined, quick-cooking grains tend to flood your neighborhood with sugars. Light fluffy breads, many breakfast cereals, and even pretzels tend to do the same. Read labels, even fruit juice labels. Be sure they are 100% pure juice, and be intelligent about the quantity you consume at one time as they can be carb heavy. Healthy carbs are most efficient and they help to "green" your neighborhood. Sweet!

Heated and depleted

As food is heated beyond its natural ambient temperature range, it takes on a new flavor, literally and energetically. As you have already learned, fats are very sensitive to heat, but proteins, carbs and all the other components of the food are also affected in their own way. Thus the more you heat, the more you "deplete" the food's *natural* energetic flavor. In fact, browning or blackening foods can produce toxic baggage that you then consume. When we use "waves of convenience" via the microwave oven to unnaturally heat food, we "push the envelope" even further and can turn it into faux-food. It is in your best interest to wave goodbye to your microwave. Your body will love you for it!

Be committed…

You have been given an abundance of food for thought about food. You can take your nutritional choices to higher and higher levels of respect as you move to avoid even the tiniest bits of negative energy that could affect your neighborhood flow. For example, do your best to avoid all chemical preservatives, unnatural food colorings, and flavor "enhancers," such as MSG and other ambiguously named isolates and extracts. You will be naturally motivated to avoid these additives as you apply the basic keys to food choices as we have discussed, so do not put any pressure on yourself to transition all at once.

If you know that your current dietary habits have been low-energy and are concerned about the availability of foods that will strengthen your neighborhood…don't panic. Fortunately, an ever increasing variety of food products are available that are free from hydrogenated oils, are labeled non-GMO, have no added salt, and are organic and not enriched. You can take baby steps to transition, but once in motion you must continue to move forward and not ever take a step back. Be aware that many packaged food wrappers, bags, and containers advertise "all natural" in big letters, while the ingredient list is in small barely readable print. "All natural" is not equivalent to "organic" nor does it mean that all the ingredients are healthy for you. Thus, do not be taken in by the advertising on the package. Just be sure to have your reading glasses with you, because you must read the ingredient lists!

Cholesterol

Before we move on, I must dispel some myths about your neighborhood cholesterol. First…*it is not bad!* Your body could not survive without it and your body even manufactures its own to be sure you have enough. Do you realize that your LDL and HDL do not represent cholesterol? They are the transport vehicles that *carry* your cholesterol around the 'hood! They are lipoproteins, and your body also could not thrive without them. Thus, there is no bad versus good argument. As you now know, the question you must ask yourself is, "So what does a true excess or deficiency *imbalance* of LDL and HDL represent?" As always, look to the natural keys. It may be a request to "get moving," i.e., optimize your intelligent aerobic exercise. It is often a request to avoid faux fats and refined carbs. It may be a request to consume more raw vegetables for natural vitamins and fiber. It may reflect a secondary effect of emotional stress energy! Are anger/hostility, guilt, and fear disturbing your neighborhood LDL and HDL balance? Yes.

On the other hand, it is *not* a request to commit to a lifetime of prescription medication. Although there are urgent and emergent situations where these have a place, including the rare occasion where one shows profound imbalance due to especially challenging genetic tendencies, the way to healthy balance lies within the natural keys. Thus, do not fear cholesterol, LDL, and HDL. Rather, if you are faced with an imbalance…just answer the question!

CHAPTER TWELVE

THE BLOOD-BRAIN BARRIER TO WORLD HEALING

Your neighborhood actually has a blood-brain barrier to protect your core – your brain – from unwanted intruders. There are three energetic influences that find their way through to throw your neurotransmitters out of balance. They are alcohol, nicotine, and caffeine. They are the most widely used brain altering substances in the world. In addition to the catastrophic amount of body dis-ease that their misuse has caused, you may not be aware that, collectively, their abuse is also significantly responsible for humanity's delay in achieving emotional maturity!

As we discussed early in the text, most of the world uses the term "stressed out" to place the "blame" for their body emotions and symptoms on what is going on outside of them. Thus, it is not surprising that people look for quick fixes outside of themselves to deal with their suppressed emotions and fear. Now that you know stress occurs within, you know that you must understand what is happening within, in order to address this misalignment! Let's discuss these energies and shatter some myths.

Alcohol

Alcohol stresses you in all over your neighborhood. Unfortunately, whatever you have heard, there is no such thing as low risk drinking, because the line between any possible benefit and the risks is individual to each person. Advertising has done its job by suggesting that it reduces heart dis-ease, and thus, it is healthy for you. Well, that is false and false. Beverages that contain alcohol may affect the incidence of dis-ease in the *blood vessels* that supply the heart and indirectly affect the incidence of vascular-related events in specific risk groups, but it is directly and indirectly toxic to your heart muscle itself! It is also toxic to your brain and many other organs including the liver; it can induce subtle or profound vitamin and mineral imbalances; and it is a risk factor for cancer, including breast cancer! These risks are well documented.

So, take your pick: Do you want healthy and pristine body organs, knowing that you will actually lower your risk of vascular dis-ease by working with all of the natural keys? Or, do you want to consume alcohol for the possibility that it may contribute to less arterial dis-ease, only to find out that, despite a holistic and organic lifestyle, your body may never be quite in balance, or you develop an alcohol-related condition such as fatty liver or more threatening dis-ease?

Thus, the first point you must understand is that **alcohol, in any form, is not a preventive care tool!** Many of you may be thinking, "Well, I can grasp the truth of that relating to harder liquor and beer, but what about grape wine…doesn't it have special substances that can help my body? Also, since wine is used in certain religious observances, wouldn't it mean that it has good energy?" Insightful questions…let's answer them one by one.

First, it is *grapes,* especially the skins, which contain naturally packaged antioxidants and other substances. Wine can contain essences of these substances, such as resveratrol, but the quality of their energies is in doubt once yeasts ferment the grapes' sugars to produce alcohol. Since there is no evidence of a net positive effect of wine on total body health, the act of drinking wine solely for the resveratrol and other substances would be like eating a raisin cookie made with partially hydrogenated oil, refined sugar, and bleached flour to possibly get health benefits from the vitamins in the raisin! Catch the drift?

As far as religious tradition and observances, did you know that the most historically prominent prayer recited "over wine" makes no mention of wine? It specifically is a loving acknowledgment of God who "creates the *fruit* of the vine." The fruit of the vine is the grape…not alcoholic wine. Thus, a sip of grape juice is often used in its place. Also, many people proceed to the altar during services in their house of worship to take a sip of wine. In both instances, the sip of the sweet juice or the fermented grape represents a spiritual connection. In other words, wine has an essence of the fruit of the vine whose building blocks ultimately trace back to a highest creative essence. Thus, it is a sacred symbol within specific religious ritual, but it is not a scriptural endorsement that consumption of alcoholic wine outside of this context is in any way healthy or necessary to achieve spiritual maturity.

I know what your next question is. "I enjoy the taste of wine. What if I drink only one half or one glass per day?" I have just one thing to say about that…your epigenome! Your personal epigenome is vulnerable to everything that enters your neighborhood. Since we do not know if there even is a minimum threshold where your epigenetic keys are turned to send your DNA down a dangerous path, it is very risky to regularly send alcohol into your neighborhood in any amount.

Be sure to completely abstain from alcohol during pregnancy. Regardless of what your physician tells you, drinking alcohol during pregnancy would be considered physical abuse of your child's body.

In fact, the key breaking the vicious cycle of alcohol use lies with children! You must share the truth with your children from an early age and also teach them by example. You must start early, because most people in the world begin to consume alcohol in their teenage years! Teenagers are not sipping a glass of wine over lunch while they discuss politics. They are drinking significant quantities of alcohol at social gatherings and, according to statistics kept even by colleges and universities themselves, they are very often binge drinking. Thus, respectfully timed discussions with children explaining that alcohol can injure their organs, delay their emotional maturity, and affect the health of their future children and grandchildren will absolutely reduce the overall incidence of alcohol use.

Also, because advertisements and commercials for alcohol are everywhere and are very well-staged, it is actually beneficial to occasionally remind them that those people are actors hired to pretend that alcohol is necessary to have an enjoyable time at a social event. Explain to them that the truth of the matter is that choosing not to drink reflects a higher degree of maturity, will lower their risk of engaging in a high risk activity that may weigh heavily on them for the rest of their lives, and their future children and grandchildren will love them for it!

One final comment: The concept that you are recovering since you released a drinking habit is false. What are you recovering from? You just didn't know how to deal naturally with your emotions, fears, and epigenetic tendencies. When you release this habit, or any other habit that is misaligned, it means that you have *matured* emotionally and/or spiritually. The reason some people return to this habit, or to using any brain-altering substance, is because when faced with new challenges or loneliness, they often reinsert fear and lose faith, which throws their body out of ease. So they look outside themselves again for a quick way to drown their emotions. Drowning your emotions will bury you. Many of you know the truth of this. Remember, your body will never send a request for you to bring alcohol into the neighborhood. Use your new foundation of knowledge to address your emotions sooner than later. Your body and everybody will love you for it.

Caffeine

I know you are saying, wait a minute, aren't there medicinal uses for caffeine? Yes, but related to *lung* function for very specific respiratory urgencies or emergencies. As far as the brain, once in a while, if you need to be more alert in an urgent or emergent situation, then it may have a place. Otherwise, used chronically, it stresses you in. Your body reminds you of this when releasing the habit, as most of you experience the discontinuation symptoms (headaches, etc.) that occur as your body works to recalibrate your neurotransmitters. Insomnia and heart palpitations, to name a few, may also be messages from your body that it is not at ease with caffeine.

The main point is that caffeine is the world's most popular brain-altering drug, and since most people will honestly admit that they drink coffee and colas specifically to "combat" fatigue and feel more awake, **much of the world is self-medicating the symptom of fatigue instead of moving to uncover the true underlying cause!** By masking your symptom, you may be delaying the discovery of potentially imminently threatening dis-ease and, because the deepest root of the fatigue symptom is very often emotional stress energy, caffeine can delay your road to emotional maturity. Know the difference between fatigue and healthy tiredness. Healthy tiredness is your complex neighborhood biological clock preparing your body to relax so that your brain can focus on generating its healing and recharging waves of sleep. This, as I mentioned earlier, occurs most naturally as sunlight fades to nightfall. Thus, the term "a good night's sleep."

In contrast, fatigue is a message from your body that it is not at ease. Thus, **you never want to "combat" fatigue, as this would mean going to war with your body!** Find out first what this message represents and deal with it appropriately. Your body perceives caffeine or sleeping pills as your attempt to muzzle its voice, and your body will find an alternate way to nudge you… other symptoms! This understanding is really important!

Whether you have fatigue or not, take a holiday from all caffeinated beverages and other sources of caffeine for a few weeks. You may or may not have obvious recalibration symptoms, but your body is working to restore harmony nonetheless. If you unmask or continue to experience any ongoing symptoms, such as fatigue or headache, then your body has other issues it wants you to address, and you need to find out what these symptoms represent and deal with them appropriately. Do not self-medicate again with caffeine! More often than not, after your physician's workup has excluded obvious causes, you will discover that emotional stress energies (worry, fear, suppressed emotions) are at the core. Fortunately, now you know how to manage this.

If you enjoy a cup of tea or coffee, intelligently reintroduce these beverages only if you do not have any unexplained symptoms! Also, allow your brain to wake up naturally in the morning before any caffeine is consumed. Never reintroduce any beverage or otherwise that lists caffeine as an added ingredient, such as many colas and soft drinks. The advertised energy boost is all negative energy from its detached caffeine and other ingredients. Also, please be aware that the intake of caffeinated beverages in pregnancy should be zero. Your baby is exposed to its effects directly and indirectly, and caffeine may be a risk factor for miscarriage.

Nicotine

Since you are well aware of the profound extent to which tobacco smoke stresses in your neighborhood, why would you knowingly disrespect your body? That's the nicotine paradox, isn't it? Now that you know your epigenome is being battered with all the toxic baggage, and that your discontinuation symptoms are your body's recalibration of neurotransmitters, you may actually be able to grin and bear the transition period this time. You will emerge with a stronger mind, and your body will love you for it. If people can quit on a dime in the face of imminent danger (e.g., heart attack), then you have no excuse not to quit.

There is one question that is especially important for you to answer to help to release the nicotine habit. That is, if you began smoking since it was revealed that smoking was harmful for you, why did you start smoking in the first place?" When you can allow your answer to stare you in the face and reflect on it, you will have a breakthrough. For example, many of you will say that you wanted to be accepted by peers or that it would make you seem cool. Is that the case now? Do you have any idea how many people have downsized their time spent with you then and now because you smoke? Of course, it's not because people don't love you; it's just that the smoke is so incredibly dissonant to most people that it is uncomfortable to spend time in that energy.

Maybe you started smoking because you heard it made you "feel good." Do you feel good now? Do you realize that you only smoke now because you are not at ease unless you do have a cigarette? It's an illusion, my friends. Your nicotine is now a band-aid to keep you treading water…that's all it does.

When you do get past the initial recalibration process, the same truth holds as with alcohol. If you experience "nervous" symptoms and your first thought is to find a cigarette, remind yourself that the symptom represents a message from your body that there is an emotion that you have not dealt with. It is never a message to throw nicotine at your neighborhood! Also, you have an obligation to teach your children that **a nicotine habit will ensure that they will never be able to feel their feelings the way they are naturally supposed to.** This statement is energetically correct. That should get their attention.

Word on the street...

The word on your neighborhood street is that "street drugs" are also brain ambushers, and they all stress you in. There are not many who would debate this. I should touch on one rather controversial substance you know as cannabis. There are still those who believe that it is safe for you. This is false. First, the smoke generated from burning anything and exposing your lungs to it has toxic baggage, as you now know. Second, researchers have discovered natural cannabis-like neuropeptides, such as anadamides, in your neighborhood with their own receptors. Thus, when you throw cannabis at your neighborhood, it crowds these receptor sites and your body must recalibrate. Thus, by definition, cannabis stresses you in. (The debate whether cannabis should be used in a hospice or palliative care setting is a topic for another place and time.)

For those who find themselves caught in the vicious cycle of these various "street drugs," first remind yourself that you are not a bad person. You are just not currently in spirit, thus you have been looking for love in all the wrong places. You are hesitant to move to release this habit because you fear that you will not like what you see when you emerge from the fog. Actually you will not like what you see...you will love what you see. You will have clarity for maybe the first time in a long time and you will reconnect with your true self. It's time to enlist someone to assist you as you safely ease away from this habit. As long as you rekindle and strengthen your individual dialogue with the highest source, you will be able to persevere as your body works to restore harmony.

"Space invaders"

As you know, our planet is now littered with the byproducts of burning fossil fuels, industrial manufacturing and refining, and spraying crops and other plant life. Some of these are natural energies, such as heavy metals that have been displaced from their naturally safe havens within the earth. Others are industry-produced toxins that always stress you in. When they gain access to your neighborhood, they take up space that has been reserved for your natural building blocks.

Let's look at the metal mercury, for example. It is a natural energy but it is not naturally supposed to be present in enough quantity to bump your neighborhood residents out of their seats. Unfortunately, we have allowed it to be injected (via vaccines) directly into our neighborhood and have also filled dental cavities with it, where it can leach into our body. In addition, many of the fish we consume have been contaminated with unnaturally high levels of mercury. From this point on, never allow a mercury amalgam filling to enter your neighborhood or the mouths of your children. There are always more respectful options for dental health.

What about other metals, chemicals, and pesticides? Yes, all of them are "space invaders" and stress you in. All sources of drinking water contain some space invaders; however, many public sources are very concerning due to the added baggage such as chlorine byproducts, added fluoride, and other invaders. Significantly limit your time in the shower whether you have a filter or not. Space invaders can breech your neighborhood via vapors and skin contact. How to provide clean drinking water unconditionally to all people on a large scale is one issue that has been swept under the rug. Since most of our neighborhood is water energy, this must be addressed. Access to clean water is a right, not a privilege.

Did you know that most food and beverage cans have an inner coating that contains a space invader called bisphenol A? Just read about the potential stress-in effects of bisphenol A and I guarantee that you will immediately begin to limit your use of these cans and, instead, look for naturally good alternatives in glass. Plastic containers can also harbor space invaders and have literally become environmental "space invaders" themselves. Did you know that there are some promising plant based alternatives to plastic on the horizon? What about cookware? Chemically coated nonstick cookware can release highly toxic space invaders when heated. Your metal pots and pans can also potentially emit space invaders. Remember that your body builds most effectively and efficiently with nature's raw or gently heated foods. Retire your nonstick chemically coated items and use your other cookware intelligently and sparingly.

You must always be aware that anything that contacts your skin can potentially be absorbed and enter your neighborhood. In fact, it is best to consider that everything you apply to your skin will be absorbed, so that you will minimize your exposure to toxic substances. Why do you need all of those cosmetics, creams, and screens, anyway?

For those of you who are excited about nanotechnology… think again. As more industry goes nano, workers and others will be exposed to these tiny particles. Nanoparticles have the potential to breach the skin of living organisms! What about inhaled nanos? Could they lodge and be another "asbestos-like" disaster waiting to happen? Since nanos may turn out to be no-no's, please be a very wary and educated observer.

Since many of the space invaders that your body works to release (i.e., naturally excrete) end up in the sludge of your local wastewater plant where, ultimately, the sludge is often returned to the land (disturbingly, often processed and repackaged under the disguise of fertilizer which is then used on farms), we clearly have a vicious cycle in place. Thus, the key to breaking this cycle does not lie in a lifelong commitment to costly maintenance body detoxification protocols with detached vitamins, supplements and chelators, as this is just riding an endless roller coaster of unclear benefit and ignoring the root of the problem.

The answer does reside in, literally, keeping our noses out of Earth's business! That is, instead of keeping our collective heads buried, looking deep beneath the Earth's surface for fuel sources, we need to look one hundred and eighty degrees in the opposite direction. In other words, we must stop drilling and mining for fuels, and start to expeditiously tap into the infinite and clean energy of the sun, wind and, of course, the higher influences. Solar cells and panels that catch the sun's photons with increasingly greater efficiency will continue to become more available. It's time!

You may be wondering how the highest influence relates to directly impacting space invaders. You already know that Love is the most healing influence for your body physiology, thus it is a fact that your natural detoxification system will also be more at ease and more efficient with love. How many of you have seen photographs of water becoming more beautifully structured and pristine after being exposed to the influence of loving words?

Whether or not this finding can be reproduced, it does bring to light important joules for thought. Since water comprises such a significant percentage of your neighborhood vibe, is it then within the realm of possibility that beautifying the mind and staying resolutely connected to love can further enhance the body's detoxification beyond what we would naturally expect?

Vaccines: what do they impart?

Vaccines are a hotly debated topic. Many are pointing fingers at vaccine components in relation to childhood syndromes such as autism. Let's examine vaccines as we have examined every other energetic influence. Almost every component of vaccines is of unnatural vibration. We see components that have been altered from their natural state (attenuated microorganisms). We see cell fragments often harvested from unlike organisms. What about the polysorbate-80, neomycin, and even traces of bovine calf serum? The most publicity had been directed at mercury, so the manufacturers woke up enough to begin to address this problem. Unfortunately, we are now stuck with aluminum in many of our vaccines! Yes, aluminum. Mercury and aluminum are very unwelcome invaders within your neighborhood nervous system and elsewhere. Yet, we send them over and over again into our babies' neighborhoods.

Pushing a sharp object through your skin's natural force field is unsettling enough to your neighborhood. Injecting space invaders directly into your neighborhood would be considered an ambush. Thus, vaccines stress you in and clearly have the potential to contribute to more serious dis-ease, and we certainly cannot say that vaccines have been a net positive influence over the course of anyone's lifetime or to humanity in general. With a few exceptions (for example, vaccination after an acute neighborhood breach such as occurs with certain penetrating wounds or a rabid animal bite), it is clearly possible that vaccines have contributed to more morbidity than would have occurred without them.

So, how do we begin to sort this out? Since childhood brain dis-ease syndromes (from subtle learning and emotional disabilities to autism) seem to have increased in the last few decades, if we want to determine if vaccines' stress-in effects have contributed to this spectrum of dis-ease, we would have to begin by not initiating specific vaccines until after children have reached certain milestones, such as after they are able to talk. Of course this would be a difficult decision for many, since most parents or guardians would insert and chronically carry fear that their child would be more vulnerable to certain infectious organisms and then insert almost catastrophic guilt if the child experienced serious body infection.

Use your new mindset and knowledge to make a decision. Now that you know what energies are contained within the vaccine cocktail, you know they do stress the neighborhood, at least to some degree. You also know that any fear carried in relation to your decision will stress in both you and your baby. Thus, whatever you decide about vaccinations, you must move on without fear or regret and stay tuned to this issue for any additional pearls of knowledge that may come to light.

Using your newly acquired keys to keep the maternal neighborhood pristine from conception to childbirth, and then ensuring a naturally healthy, breast-fed and loving ambient environment for the baby would be a good start.

CHAPTER THIRTEEN

MY DOCTOR SAID...

*E*ver*y* mankind-produced pharmaceutical drug stresses you in. Reported side-effects are only the tip of the iceberg of the actual incidence of body dis-ease that they cause. With physician prescribed medication, apply the same due diligence that you have learned regarding supplements. If you have an urgent/emergent situation, then the low energy in the vial can support your neighborhood for a short while. With certain chronic states of dis-ease, such as when your pancreas can no longer produce insulin, as in type 1 diabetes, then you are taking insulin in a bottle to literally save your physical life. If your thyroid gland has been damaged and is not functioning, then thyroid in a bottle is clearly necessary. These and other specific types of situations tip the risk/benefit ratio to where you must choose the low energy (in the medicine bottle) to avoid the possibility of "no energy" (the collapse of your neighborhood).

If you reside at a geographical latitude where you cannot receive adequate exposure to the Sun's ultraviolet waves during the fall and winter, and since sunny hormone D is so vitally important to your neighborhood, then hormone D in a bottle (which does not require a prescription) may have enough useful energy to support your immune system through these months.

In general, however, the majority of pharmaceutical drugs are chemical foreigners to your neighborhood and are manufactured to suppress symptoms, block receptor sites, inhibit enzymes, and destroy microorganisms. Again, for life's urgencies and emergencies they have a place. Otherwise, used chronically, they will keep you from realizing your highest and best potential. When a critical mass of people apply the keys to wellness presented in the text, there will be a dramatic decrease in the incidence of chronic dis-ease and medication use, which will eliminate our healthcare crisis in a relatively short period of time. This is not speculation. It is evidence based on the fact that the overwhelming majority of physician hours and healthcare monetary resources are used to "treat" chronic dis-ease, to treat the secondary dis-ease emergencies that are the result of the chronic dis-ease, and to address the side effects from the medication used to treat the chronic dis-ease!

If you are already on chronic medication, never abruptly discontinue any of them and never wean them without the watchful eye of the practitioner who prescribed them. However, *do always* use your newly acquired abundance of knowledge to continually reassess your need for medication. You will find that you can almost always at least streamline your personal "polypharmacy" to a knowledge-based minimum.

A word about "over the counter" drugs: OTC does not stand for Ok To Consume. Aspirin, acetaminophen, ibuprofen, and others all stress you in. For specific urgencies and emergencies they have a place. Otherwise, be very careful before you go down the path of self-medication to suppress your symptoms. You may be wondering about aspirin, the substance that has, at times, been referred to as the wonder drug. First, there are no wonder drugs. Second, you may have been led to believe that an aspirin a day will keep the cardiologist away. This is a false generalization.

If you had previously experienced symptoms or consequences of cardiovascular dis-ease, then an aspirin a day may assist you along the way…until you apply the true keys to address the dis-ease! Otherwise, for people who are fully committed to a natural knowledge-based approach to minimize all risk factors for body dis-ease, aspirin taken chronically may present more risks than benefits, including the possibility of physically life-threatening dis-ease.

Here is some knowledge that will allow many of you to take a quantum leap along the learning curve. For the millions of you diagnosed with the symptom complex labeled irritable bowel syndrome, you must understand that your bowel symptoms are not your body's request to chronically take laxatives, anti-motility drugs, acid blockers, antibiotics, or tranquilizers. The major keys to easing these symptoms to a manageable state are found within this text, especially in the realm of emotional energy management. I am sure that almost all of you can sense the truth of this. There will soon be an ever increasing number of practitioners who become facilitators of knowledge regarding the intricacies of the keys presented in this text and who can guide you objectively as your symptoms ease.

For those of you given a diagnosis of fibromyalgia syndrome, please understand that your pain symptoms are not your body's request for narcotics or neurotransmitter-affecting drugs. Emotional energy management is also your key to easing fibromyalgia symptoms and decreasing your medication. You actually may find it more of a challenge to wean yourself off the pain medication than to naturally ease your pain symptoms! That is why it is so important not to initiate narcotic medication when you are first diagnosed.

Chronic fatigue syndrome is in the same realm. Your fatigue is not a request for caffeine, stimulant medication, or excessive sleeping hours. The fatigue of this syndrome can be totally eased with pure knowledge of the major keys and their application to your life ongoing. This is not speculation.

Again, in the future more practitioners will be available who understand stress energy and can guide you with objectivity and compassion.

Depression symptoms often surface when struggling with the three aforementioned syndromes. As you will soon learn, the major key to easing depression symptoms resides within the higher influences!

If you are diagnosed with an insidious condition such as hypertension or non-insulin dependent diabetes, then, even if you initially "require" medication, you should know that applying the keys within the text will give you a significant chance of reducing your medication or weaning off of it all together. What about the more inflammatory states of chronic dis-ease, such as those classified as auto-immune conditions? Remember that your immune system is exquisitely sensitive to stress energy. Connecting the dots on these complex dis-ease conditions is more complex, but there is a combination of keys for you as a unique individual.

Since you do not know how close your epigenome is to changing its tune in your favor, you must optimize all of the keys within the text! The next natural step you take could flip the switch. Even those with deeply stressed-in islands of cells known as cancer still have the potential to epigenetically influence the course of this dis-ease.

Anxiety and depression symptoms: what do they represent?

Since anxiety and depression symptoms are linked to so many conditions, and the medications for these are usually seen near the top of the most prescribed list, I will review them in terms that you now understand.

When you are experiencing chronic anxiety symptoms, energetically, this means you have kept your mind's worry and fear record turned on, which, for most of you, has led to the accumulation of years of stuffed body emotions. In addition, many of you may have allowed unresolved issues to pile up, so your space has become energetically cluttered and you have become overwhelmed. Think of all of the pins on your neighborhood hypothalamus that we know and love. Fear also keeps you in the "what if" game that tends to take your mind to the worst possible scenario instead of looking forward to the best.

As you learned earlier, the complex of symptoms of anxiety is one of the earliest messages from your body that it is not at ease. This can begin very early in childhood, as many can relate. If your body's message is not addressed, as you now know, your body may have to send a second wave of guiding symptoms to get your attention. Let's remove some pins for you right now!

First, for those of you playing the "What if something bad happens" game, you need to understand how this is stressing you in. The most prevalent example of this may well involve inserting worry and fear about your kids. How many of you are in this category or know somebody who is chronically stressed-in due to worry about their children? Although we absolutely have an obligation to look out for their safety and guide them responsibly, we are not meant to chronically worry or insert fear that something bad will happen along their life's path if we don't micromanage their life. The fact is, micromanaging your child's life path is equivalent to you spinning a web outside of the natural fabric. Since it will be your web that your child is forced to navigate, you will be more prone to insert guilt every time a challenge arises. This leads to more fear and micromanagement, and even to your directing anger at others. This vicious cycle stresses you in and it slows your child's path to emotional maturity.

On the other end of the spectrum, many of you may insert fear that if you do not give in to everything that your child wants or wants to do, then they will not love you. This is false and this will also delay their emotional maturity. It is neither management nor free rein that they need...it is guidance. That is, knowledge-based guidance with honest communication as you emphasize the benefits of making respectful choices. Then, as you choose to look forward to the best, every body will be more at ease.

For those of you who tend chronically to sweep your everyday chores or responsibilities under the rug, please remember that they will all become pins on your hypothalamus which will contribute to anxiety symptoms. This is another form of clutter dissonance, and another time when you should be m.a.d. Make a decision to lift up this rug and make a list (a discovery list, not a fear list) of everything you find there. It may not be a pretty sight, but I guarantee that it will become more of a tangled web if you leave it. This will give you the opportunity to take inventory of the time and resources required to remove the pins so that you can set a plan in motion to maintain a healthy daily net balance of good energy as you shorten this list.

For those of you who have a neighborhood stuffed with years of revealing emotions because you were afraid to express your honest feelings, you will be happy to know that you do not have to release them one by one! Here is a metaphor that will explain this energetically. Many of you relate that, as a child, your honest expressions, responses, or genuine efforts were always met with lean-spirited laughter or comments such as, "You don't know what you're talking about," "That's not right," "That's not good enough," "Only speak when spoken to," or other comments that may have induced you to insert fear or guilt. Let's say you internalized emotions from one parent in particular, over and over again. It is very likely that this is one of the factors that is contributing to your chronic anxiety symptoms or other symptoms of energy imbalance.

Picture each of these stuffed emotions as identical red spheres or balls. See them in a container of identical balls. The container has a round opening for the balls to flow through, and after the first rolls out, the rest can all follow. Even though you can't return to the past to release these "spheres" of emotional stress energy, if you create an "opening," the next time you have the opportunity to respond with compassionate release as you field the energy of yet another lean-spirited remark from your loved one, the entire identical group of spheres from the past has the opportunity to be released along with it.

Since many people report a rather dramatic easing of symptoms relating to that particular person after using the proper keys just once, we know that the metaphor is accurate. Otherwise, if you added energy to an already stuffed space and then released only the energy that just entered, there would be no net change in vibration and no easing of symptoms!

In addition, since you have now learned to communicate without anger or resentment, metaphorically the spheres will cycle out "green" as you are easing your neighborhood and helping to awaken the sleeper. Remember not to insert fear about what the person might say or do in response. Unless you have reason to believe that the person will respond with physical violence, you now know that compassionate release results in clarity on many levels. Remember that their choices and responses do not define your happiness. *You* can still generate loving influences towards them even if they insert anger and choose to distance themselves!

The physiology of chronic depression still remains quite a mystery to researchers. Now that the epigenome has entered the picture, we may now have a better idea as to why certain tendencies to have depression symptoms seem to cluster in families. Even though medication for depression may currently be among the most frequently prescribed medication in the United States, clinicians are quietly wondering what is exactly happening in your brain. Why are the "intended" effects of the medication so inconsistent, yet the side-effects are so prevalent and persistent? And why do some of these medications also tamper with your anxiety symptoms?

It seems as though our new best friend, the hypothalamus, is entering the picture again! In fact, a neuropeptide that your hypothalamus secretes, a hormone called CRF, now seems to be entering the spotlight of research in the realm of depression. Interestingly, CRF and receptors for CRF are also found in other areas of the emotional brain, including, do I dare say, the hippocampus! One thing should now be clear to you. That is, chronically suppressing or muzzling your body's voice as it sends symptoms will barely keep you treading water energetically.

When experiencing chronic depression symptoms, the first step is to avoid saying, "I'm depressed." You are not! You have depression *symptoms.* Saying you are depressed paints a picture that there is something outside your body that is compressing your body in some way. If a doctor says you are depressed, please clarify that you may have depression symptoms, but that you are not depressed. When they respond, "What's the difference?" you can enlighten them with your knowledge.

The next step, as you now know, is to ask yourself what your symptoms represent. If you adopt the mindset that your depression symptoms represent a genetic barrier without keys and that you are destined to a life of prescription medication or neurotransmitter supplements, your body will never be at ease. Yes, inherited epigenetic influences may make it more of a challenge for you to see the light, but the proper foundation of knowledge will dissolve these challenges. Remember that your epigenome always has the potential to change its tune in your favor.

Many people use the words "sadness" and "depression" interchangeably. This is not accurate. Understanding where sadness ends and where depression symptoms begin will make all the difference in the world. They do have something in common. That is, they both represent a shift in the balance of loving influences. Beyond that, however, there is a world of difference energetically.

Consider sadness to be your body's response to a distancing from or a passing of one who has contributed or represented loving influences along your life's path, or your empathic response to others who appear to be struggling profoundly and are literally crying out for loving influences. In essence, it is the physiology of grieving. The most profound is the passing of a loved one. Since there are no vacuums or empty spaces energetically within your body, something must come in to fill this sudden relative decrease in loving influences.

What do you think would be most appropriate and soothing to your body to ease you through this time? Of course, that would be other sources of loving influences. Fortunately, this generally happens, as others show up to offer love and support as you are grieving. Although it is understood that you cannot replace the uniqueness of the departed loved one, as long as you maintain a sense of purpose, a strong connection with the highest essence and an understanding that the Divine essence of your loved one has been displaced…but not erased…then your sadness can ease over time to a level of loving remembrance.

The road to depression symptoms occurs when we choose to replace loving influences with negative energetic influences, or we become distanced from other loving influences. What would you expect to happen when you try to fill a place within you previously occupied by loving influences with fear, guilt, and/or anger? You would develop a mindset of hopelessness, uselessness, and/or helplessness. Is it any wonder that you lose interest in activities and hobbies that you previously found enjoyable? That should be a strong message that there are other influences that need to come into your space.

When you acknowledge the facts that...

> 1) your life is and can always be purposeful (your soul's essence), despite even the most difficult challenges. You do make a difference!
>
> 2) when you address your fear, guilt, and anger, and set good purposeful thought energy-in-motion, synchronicity will always bring you in touch with loving companions; you have hope!
>
> 3) a humble and respectful connection with the highest essence will bring ease and carry you through the most challenging times; you have help!

...then your body will respond in kind physiologically and you can feel joy as you are meant to experience it.

Here are some examples to reflect upon:

> 1) A man relates that he has experienced a lifelong history of depression and anxiety symptoms, but he has resisted recommendations to start prescription medication because he was awake to the slippery slope that medication could cause. Alternatively, he has spent years attempting to balance his neighborhood physiology with supplements and rigid dietary guidelines. He was "sure" that if he could just fight those sugar cravings he would be okay. When asked the proper questions, he revealed many clues. He stated that he had friends but being with them didn't ease his symptoms. Hobbies that he would normally enjoy also did not bring ease. He had a sense of good purpose, wanting to be in the health and healing field, but he inserted fear that he would

not find his niche. He believed in a higher influence, but the nature of synchronicity had never been shared with him. He revealed that he had only ever once been involved in a closely bonded adult relationship, but that also was the one time when his body truly felt at ease. Now that's a major clue! He was of the mindset that he would only look attractive if he maintained a strict diet, but even then he had little hope that he could meet someone.

The moment he came to an understanding that the path to his closely bonded loving relationship must begin with the acknowledgment that he can and absolutely will meet that person as he places in motion an abundance of thought energy towards this desire, you could physically see his facial expression and body ease as this "light" went on in his head. Just the inner acknowledgment that he now understood one of the messages behind the symptoms caused a clear body response! He also understood that when this relationship does manifest, he should expect his symptoms to ease even further. When he is able to acknowledge that sugar cravings and food concerns are band-aids and red herrings, and that his friends and hobbies fill a different energetic niche for his body, he should expect to feel more at ease with these friendships, as he now recognizes what they do and do not represent.

2) A woman past child-bearing age relates chronic depression symptoms. She is married and does not presently describe this as loving companionship, but she is afraid to dialogue in truth to determine if a truly significant relation-drift had occurred. Her job environment was extremely dissonant due to an

abundance of lean-spirited words and actions coming from her employers, but she was afraid to respond to her emotions. She had lost her sense of purpose. In the past, she had made a fear-based decision to end a pregnancy and she never carried any children to term. She inserted catastrophic guilt due to this. She held lifelong anger towards her mother, and stuffed tons of emotional energy within this relationship. She had lost a close relative a few years earlier. She believed in a higher influence, but she appeared to have a faint current of thought that, because of her past choices and actions, she may somehow now "not be in favor" with the highest essence which, of course, could not be further from the truth.

When asked when her body had felt most at ease, she related that, despite the fear and lack of parental emotional support, when she was carrying the children within her womb, she would feel a sense of loving influences from within. She also had ease when thinking about working with people in a healing capacity. Not surprisingly, this person also had been diagnosed with symptoms of chronic fatigue and fibromyalgia syndromes, and it was clear that she desperately needed to use the appropriate keys to create space through the release of all the emotional energy that was generated or stuffed within.

Regarding her depression symptoms, she felt noticeably "lighter" as she grasped the truth that they did represent a physiologic yearning for loving influences and that *she* actually held keys that would increase the flow of loving influences coming into her neighborhood. She also expressed ease the moment she came to an understanding that strengthening her spiritual connection could give her the opportunity to dissolve catastrophic guilt. She was reminded that synchronicity will always create a path for her to work her passion as long as she rekindles her sense of good purpose and sets these desires in motion without inserting fear. A lot of keys to set into motion, but all within her grasp.

3) For those of you who have a very difficult time maintaining a sense of purpose because you are faced with the difficult challenges of catastrophic bodily injury or structurally disruptive body dis-ease, please remember that as long as you have the ability to think and generate positive energetic thoughts and loving influences, you are contributing healing energy to everyone on the planet. Remember... energetically everyone is connected. As challenging as it is for one faced with these situations to release the negative influences of fear, guilt, and anger, it is vitally important to do this and to maintain a strong connection to the highest essence. You are not excluded from synchronicity and you still have the opportunity to manifest a level of healing that is beyond the limited expectations described within current medical literature!

Depression symptoms will also occur for the strongly dependent among us if they are deprived of our loving influences. Babies and very young children will become irritable and will not thrive if those who are caring for them do not lovingly hold and hug them and otherwise generate loving influences. Many of the elderly among us, when faced with multiple sensory and memory deficits, are especially vulnerable to depression symptoms if neglected or distanced from loving influences. In this population, irritability/anxiety symptoms also are usually a tip-off to underlying depression symptoms. The same is true for any emotionally and spiritually immature dependent person who cannot easily grasp the concepts of purposefulness or spiritual connectivity.

There are many people of all ages who, as they experience ever deepening depression symptoms, are falling through the cracks of societal and parental denial, fear, and even indifference. Thus, although they are literally crying out for loving influences, people with depression symptoms often only appear on the radar screen of the current healthcare system when their minds have moved to a state where their decisions can be imminently threatening to their physical lives. This is one of the major reasons we must strive to consistently shower our children with love and knowledge. Even as the pre-teen and teen experiences a natural hormonal shift, courtesy of, yes, the hypothalamus, they do listen and reflect more than they have been given credit for. So please dialogue and share knowledge about our energetic nature and the higher influences with your child from an early age. Instead of having yet another fear-based discussion about the pitfalls of parties and peer pressure, you should emphasize the perks of patience, perseverance, purpose, personal prayer, and a passion to preserve the pristine state of the neighborhood, so they can build a solid foundation of health for themselves and for their progeny. Do not try to read the preceding sentence ten times fast, but please do read it several times until it becomes a permanent resident of your neighborhood campus!

CHAPTER FOURTEEN

WE ARE ALL MENTORS AND STUDENTS

As the knowledge that has been presented within the text is applied, there will be a dramatic shift of energy in our favor. You now know that everything does matter. You now know that your thoughts, words, actions, and every joule of energy that you are exposed to molds your epigenome during your life ongoing, and these energies can hinder or optimize your future generations. That makes it even more vital that our children's emotional and spiritual learning curves reach certain milestones ahead of what society has defined thus far. Children can grasp and handle it because we are sharing knowledge, not a databank of information.

Remember, as adults, you must first open your own mind, look within and be honest with yourself about any imbalances that you need to address, because as well as sharing knowledge, you also must teach by good consistent example! In fact, every one of us on Earth has a lifelong obligation to teach and also be a respectful student. In other words, we are obligated to mentor and inspire others who have less knowledge than we do, and to be students of others that we identify as having wisdom beyond our own. This is at the core of our purpose.

For those who strive to attain a position of elected "official," please be aware that you will be stepping into the sticky web known as the political arena. Why is it that we find so few in this arena who become catalysts for positive change?

The main reason is that most people in these positions have become catalysts for "loose" change, so to speak. In other words, they consistently use a lack of monetary resources as an excuse for not being able to place purposeful policies in motion. It doesn't work that way, my friends. It has never worked and is clearly not working in the present day. Money is the red herring of all red herrings and has no place in the equation of composing a benevolent policy. Do you think that a passionate musician would make the excuse that he/she cannot compose a deeply inspired symphony because he or she is worried that there may not be an orchestra to play it? You should now understand that a truly purposeful plan will "find" a way to be successfully set in motion.

Instead of people trying to please all of the people all of the time, we need catalysts who have the backbone to *help* all the people all the time. For you as an elected official, for example, fear and greed will always move you to cater to the ungenerous mind when you should be fostering an environment that cultivates and encourages the beautiful mind of each individual. So, please, stop draining all of your energy lobbying for loose change...it will never add up to anything.

For example, begin by assembling bright and compassionate minds to compose a blueprint for health care that provides for life's urgencies and emergencies, and establishes access to ongoing knowledge for healing to dramatically reduce the incidence of chronic dis-ease. A good purposeful knowledge-based plan will pay itself back in jewels and joules many times over.

People campaigning for elected office often use the word "change." The question remains, once elected, can they be courageous enough to be resolutely committed to the role as a catalyst for positive change, or will their tenure be just another red herring? It's time that all of the world's elected officials awaken to the fact that they are on the same staircase of humanity as everybody else, and they are not immune to the consequences of disingenuous words or ungenerous actions. Even if they continue to struggle, a truly historic paradigm shift is in motion. The positive momentum cannot be altered, because a new wave of benevolence is on the horizon and is poised to awaken any elected or corporate sleepwalkers.

CHAPTER FIFTEEN

WELCOME HOME

Your journey has now come full circle, except that you have acquired an abundance of knowledge along the way, and you now stand ready to move forward to realize your highest and best potential. From the beginning of the text you learned that your quarks and electrons are perfect. They never get sick. Thus, you never get "sick" and you should never use this word to describe yourself, because it is energetically negative. Rather, your body is at ease or not at ease. There is a beautiful song that relates, "From a distance…there is…no dis-ease." It is now time to bring about a world where, at arm's length, there is no chronic dis-ease.

The coming decade will be ushered in by a necessary shift in how we achieve a true state of wellness. We don't need to have "conventional" versus "alternative" labels for health care. We *do* need all practitioners of the healing and restorative arts to become "fluent" in the true energetic nature of our body language. Stress energy management, the physiology of true spirituality, an understanding of the epigenome, and the downfall of the poly-pharmacy/poly-supplement mindset will result in a quantum leap towards Health on Earth.

You now know that everything matters and every joule of energy that you generate makes a difference in the ambient energy of the planet. The present ambient energy is tipped to the unfavorable side, but every scale can tip the other way. Since we do not know the critical mass necessary to tip the scale in our favor, it is vital that each person strive to reflect a beautiful mind with its expanding ripple of positive energetic influences.

Aside from your personal method of dialogue and prayer, two simple, yet profound additions that will add good energy are as follows: Think of S.H.I.N.E. as an acronym for **S**how **H**umanity **I**ts **N**ew **E**nergy. If you simply think or say, "rise and shine," when you arise each morning, you will reinforce your commitment to contribute to the shift towards Health on Earth. Then in the evening, when so many of you may be wrestling with a mind full of worry and fear, instead generate a simple dialogue out to the universe asking for Love and Knowledge to come through as you sleep so that you can provide the same for others the following day and every day. I guarantee the world will love you for that.

Good energy to all…and to all a good life!

ACKNOWLEDGMENTS

I would like to acknowledge everyone who has shared their love and knowledge along my life's path. I am grateful for all of you.

ABOUT THE AUTHOR

Dr. Bornstein is a holistically educated physician with over twenty-five years of patient care experience in the field of internal medicine. He has moved beyond "conventional" medicine to follow a passion, which is to be a catalyst for the necessary paradigm shift in how we approach health and wellness. He is one of an emerging group of healthcare professionals who recognize that we can significantly impact the incidence of chronic dis-ease in our lifetimes.

In teaching others how to identify their personal keys to optimal wellness, Dr. Bornstein has seen that the symptoms of many of the most prevalent and challenging conditions and syndromes can be naturally eased to restore a state of wellness. This is especially profound when we consider that many of these conditions continue to baffle the conventional medical community. Notable examples include the syndromes of chronic fatigue, fibromyalgia, and irritable bowel, as well as chronic depression symptoms.

Through private sessions, he provides education to those who are motivated to learn how they can help themselves to heal and become less dependent on the current healthcare system. Dr. Bornstein also offers continuing medical education to physicians and other practitioners of the healing arts to enhance their understanding of stress and how it relates to patient care within their specific areas of expertise.

www.ingramcontent.com/pod-product-compliance
Lightning Source LLC
Chambersburg PA
CBHW062215080426
42734CB00010B/1903